D1231736

Also by Ted Schwarz:
THE FIVE OF ME

TELL ME WHO I AM
BEFORE I DIE

TELL ME
WHO I AM
BEFORE
I DIE

Christina Peters
with Ted Schwarz_____

Rawson Associates Publishers, Inc.
New York_____

Library of Congress Cataloging in Publication Data

Peters, Christina, 1942–
Tell me who I am before I die.

1. Multiple personality—United States—Biography.
2. Peters, Christina, 1942–   I.   Schwarz,
   Theodore, joint author.   II.   Title.
RC569.5.M8P47   616.8'523 [B]   78-54689
                ISBN 0-89256-063-0

Published simultaneously in Canada by
McClelland and Stewart, Ltd.
Manufactured in the United States of America
by The Book Press, Inc., Brattleboro, Vermont
Designed by Joyce Weston
First Edition

Dedicated to those whom God hath healed

All the names in this book have been changed to protect the rights of privacy of certain individuals.

CONTENTS

Prologue 3

1   The Death of Christina 11

2   Daddy Ben and Poverty—The Early Years 26

3   Growing Apart 47

4   Adolescent Madness 55

5   Wedding-Bell Blues 77

6   Men and Madness 93

7   Personality Conflicts 112

8   Locked Up Inside 132

9   Coming Apart 142

10   Coming Together 164

11   Christina 208

TELL ME WHO I AM
BEFORE I DIE

PROLOGUE

Marie walked slowly past the liquor store, her yellowed, bloodshot eyes caressing the bottles on display in the window with a loving fondness. All her "friends" were there—Chivas Regal Scotch, Tanqueray Gin, Finlandia Vodka, Seagram's Crown Royal, Amaretto di Saronno, Heineken Lager Beer, and, of course, the cheap wine you could buy by the gallon. It was the wine she usually drank these days, not because her taste wasn't more sophisticated but rather because you got more for your money. There wasn't much kick in a half pint of the most expensive Scotch. But for the same price you could buy a couple of gallons of cheap domestic wine and forget all your troubles.

Marie's mouth felt dry and her body craved the burning warmth of the liquid the bottles contained. She lusted for a drink, her desire stronger than any she had ever felt for a man.

For the fifth time in as many minutes Marie checked her purse for money. She had found a penny in the torn lining and a dime wedged between some pictures in her wallet. But eleven cents wouldn't even buy a sip of the cheapest "Sneaky Pete." She tore the lining further, feeling the material carefully as she worked. She shook out her handkerchief, then carefully ripped a spare pair of panty hose she carried, hoping a coin might have caught in the fabric. It was useless. She didn't have the money she needed.

A loose brick in the alley at the side of the liquor store caught Marie's attention. The display window glass was protected by sensing foil which triggered an alarm when disturbed,

though it wasn't otherwise reinforced. Marie knew from past
experience how easy it would be to smash the window, grab
a bottle, and run. The trouble was that it was mid-afternoon.
A store clerk might stop her before she had a chance to get
a drink. After all, the last time she had burglarized a liquor
store the cops arrested her within minutes. She probably
wouldn't have that long this time, and if she couldn't consume
a pint or two, it wasn't worth the hassle of going to jail.

Marie took one last look at the window, then reluctantly
continued toward home. Maybe there was money in one of the
dresser drawers. Len had gotten rid of all the liquor and wine
in the house but he usually left some cash lying around. She
could buy herself all the "friends" she needed with Len's
money. He'd probably beat her for doing it if he caught her
drunk again, but what the hell . . . By then she wouldn't care.

The house was empty when Marie arrived. Len was at
work and Tina was still in school. She went immediately to
the bedroom, checking the top of the dresser first and then the
drawers. Her face was flushed and sweating. Her stomach was
beginning to cramp. The money, if it was there, was hidden.
Marie began removing clothing from the drawers—first carefully, then faster and faster until she was throwing shirts, underwear, socks, and handkerchiefs onto the floor. The cramps
were getting worse.

The bathroom! That mouthwash Len used to buy had
alcohol in it. Maybe there was some left.

Marie searched the medicine chest, then the cabinet below the sink. Len must have gotten rid of the mouthwash
after the last time he caught her drinking it. But he had left
some other "treats." His bottle of after-shave lotion had alcohol listed as one of the main ingredients. How bad could
it be?

Marie's hands were shaking as she unscrewed the top to
the after-shave lotion bottle. She took a cup, poured a little
into it, then held it beneath her nose, sniffing for a minute. It

wasn't champagne but it didn't smell bad either. She took a sip, then quickly swallowed the rest. She started to pour another cupful, paused, brought the bottle to her lips, and drained it. The alcohol in the after-shave had a calming effect.

It was obvious Len's money wasn't where he usually left it.

Tina! That was the answer. Tina got an allowance every week and Len made her save a little of it in a bank she kept in her room. He told her he didn't want her to be as stupid about money as her mother, the bastard!

Marie went into her daughter's room. She found the large glass piggy bank on a shelf in the closet. It was filled with nickels, dimes, and pennies—money Tina had saved from her allowance or earned raking leaves, washing cars, picking up her room, or just looking adorable when company came. Tina's life savings, just waiting for an emergency, and Jesus God, this was an emergency, thought Marie.

Marie took the piggy bank into the living room, turned it upside down, and began twisting and shaking it. A dime dropped through the slot in the pig's back, then another one. Five pennies were next, but the nickel which followed hit the slot at an odd angle and became wedged against some other coins. Even if she could get it loose, shaking the damn money out was going to take forever.

There was a hammer in Len's toolbox. Marie got it, came back in the living room, and struck the bank. Glass and coins flew everywhere, several slivers cutting her hands. It didn't matter.

The cramps were coming back as Marie shoved the coins into her purse. She remembered seeing a half-filled bottle of rubbing alcohol in the bathroom and went back to get it.

The clerk at the liquor store smiled at Marie. "Going to have a party?" he said, taking her money for the two gallon jugs of wine she held in her hands. He had seen her type before—once-respectable women who lived their lives in a drunken stupor. Their faces were lined, their eyes hardened. They always looked as though they had seen too much of life in too short a time and been overwhelmed by it.

Marie took the gallon jugs and walked a block to a large vacant lot that was flush against the parking lot of a major shopping center. She sat down on the ground, her feet stretched out at an angle, the jugs sitting in the V of her legs. She removed the top from one of the jugs and, with shaking hands, raised the container to her lips. She took swallow after swallow, never tasting the liquid, never feeling the sensation as it burned its way to her stomach. She continued swallowing until she needed air.

The first gallon jug was emptied in an hour. She was feeling pretty good and there was still the second jug to consume.

Maybe I should go over to Al's house, thought Marie. Al was her brother and he always left the back door of his place unlocked. She could finish the second jug there, then take a nap and not return home until she was sober.

Al's house was only two blocks away but it took Marie the better part of the next hour to reach it. She kept taking wrong turns and had to stop every few yards to satisfy her thirst. Some kids on bicycles went racing past, yelling at her and almost making her drop the wine. She cursed them, throwing a rock at them as they turned a corner and disappeared down the next street.

Marie's stomach was queasy by the time she reached Al's house. The second gallon of wine was less than half full so she put the jug to her lips and drained the remaining liquid.

The nausea grew worse. Food and liquid rose in her throat. She started to rise, then began to retch. The undigested food was spewed across the coffee table and onto the floor. She heaved and heaved, her body shaking violently each time. When she finally stopped, she slipped to the floor, her face pressed against the vomit-soaked carpet.

My wine! she thought to herself, her eyes barely focusing on the thick, foul-smelling liquid. All my wine is gone. She forced her head up slightly and studied the vomit. In the back of her mind she was remembering something she had learned in nursing school. When you regurgitate liquor, the vomit has a high alcohol content. She grabbed a vase from the table, dumped the flowers and used the bowl to try and save the noxious liquid seeping slowly into the carpet.

It won't be a total waste, Marie told herself. She could drink it again. She could . . .

It was too late. Marie lost consciousness.

Marie's first awareness was of pain. Her eyes felt as if someone was pressing his thumbs against the retinas, trying to push them back into her skull. Her head throbbed as though searing jolts of lightning were causing violent explosions in her skull.

She opened one eye, then shut it quickly. The glare of fluorescent light reflected from the bleached white pillow overwhelmed her, increasing the pain in her head. At least she knew she was in bed, though whether in her brother's home or somewhere else was still a mystery.

Minutes passed as Marie tried to adjust to the brightness enough to open her eyes and look around. Finally she forced herself to look about her.

The room, painted white, was equipped with two beds and a small table. It was an institutional setting she had seen both as a nurse and as a patient.

Marie attempted to focus her thoughts on what had happened that day. Gradually she remembered the drunken binge and her effort to save her own vomit so she wouldn't lose the alcohol. The idea shocked and sickened her.

My God, thought Marie. How low can a human being sink in this world?

Marie's mind filled with other images. She looked at her

partially paralyzed, heavily scarred left arm, remembering the times she had found herself in the hospital, healing from what everyone said was a suicide attempt. Yet she never remembered slashing her body or taking the pills the doctors said she had. She never remembered much of anything—hours, days, and even weeks of her life totally missing from her memory over the years.

I'm insane, she thought. How else can someone be alive yet not remember their existence? It wasn't the alcohol that caused her problems. It was something else, something far more serious that had forced her to live in hell long before it was time to die.

Marie thought of her family. Relations with Len had been strained for months, but Tina . . . God, how she loved that child. She had abandoned all the others. But not Tina. She wanted to make things right for that girl. Yet what good could she do for the child as long as her life was an endless nightmare of lost experiences? Tina was approaching adolescence and needed a woman's guidance to help her through her time of sexual awakening. But Marie could never be that woman so long as she continued the way she was living. All she could do was cause her child pain and sadness.

I've got to find someone . . . Get help . . . thought Marie, attempting to stand. Her legs were almost useless. Her knees buckled as though held together by a weakened hinge. She fell to the floor and began crawling to the door. She had to get a nurse, a doctor, someone . . . Someone had to help her. Someone had to bring her out of this nightmare existence so she could be a normal woman and a real mother to her daughter.

The corridor outside Marie's door was empty when she reached it. Most of the patients were either in group therapy or mindlessly watching one of the game shows on the television set in the recreation area.

Using the door for support, Marie tried to pull herself

upright. She rose to her knees, then painfully tried to stand. Her hair, cleaned by the nurses after her arrival, hung limply about her head and over her eyes. Her face, the color of chalk, was covered with perspiration. Her hospital gown was disheveled and torn from crawling. Her mouth was open, saliva trickling down her chin as she breathed rapidly. Tears filled her reddened eyes. She pulled herself erect, then leaned against the door frame as footsteps echoed in the distance. Someone was coming down the hall.

The corridor lights were even brighter than those in the room. Marie had to squint to see who was approaching. It was a man—tall, somewhat overweight, his hair uncombed and the stubble of a beard on his chin. There were deep circles under his eyes and he appeared to have been awake all night.

As the man came nearer, Marie saw it was a psychiatrist, Dr. Brewster. She had met him twice in the past. The first time was when she was in the same ward for attempting a suicide she couldn't remember. The second time he had been assigned to give her a psychiatric evaluation so a judge would know whether to send her to jail or a mental hospital for crimes she didn't remember committing. Each time she had instinctively trusted him, even though his appearance was such that he looked more like a clumsy bear than a doctor of medicine.

Dr. Brewster nodded to Marie but didn't slacken his pace. He had spent the night with a suicidal patient and he was on his way home. His office secretary had rescheduled his appointments so he could get a couple hours' rest before starting his regular work day. He had no interest in engaging in small talk with a mental patient he knew had resisted all past efforts to help her.

"Dr. Brewster," whispered Marie. Her voice sounded as though she was trying to say his name through a mouthful of gravel. She choked on the words, coughing and beginning to cry. There was so much she wanted to explain and so many questions needing answers. She felt as though this was her last chance to grab at sanity and she couldn't seem to find the right words. "Dr. Brewster . . . Help me."

The psychiatrist stopped and walked over to where Marie was leaning against the door. He took her arm and helped her back into the room. As he eased her to a sitting position, he said, "I'll try."

Perhaps Marie never would have made her request to Dr. Brewster had she known that in order to cure her he would have to take her life. Marie was not the whole person she believed herself to be. She was one of several unique individuals who dwelled within my brain. The real me, Christina, was buried so deeply in the subconscious that I had never experienced almost thirty years of my body's existence. Instead, Marie, Linda, Charlene, and the other fragments of my mind led quite separate lives, taking control of my body for whatever periods they could. You see, as Dr. Brewster was soon to discover, I was the victim of one of the most shocking and unusual forms of insanity known to man. I was a multiple personality.

1

THE DEATH OF CHRISTINA

As I was eventually to learn from Dr. Brewster, multiple personality cases are unusual but not rare. The first truly extensive study of a multiple personality was made by Dr. Morton Prince shortly after the turn of the century. He published a book entitled *The Dissociation of a Personality* which was the story of a multiple personality patient he studied but did not cure during the last years of his life. More recently there have been such popular books as *The Three Faces of Eve*, later made into an Academy Award winning movie, *Sybil*, which brought the problem to television, and *The Five of Me*, the first book by a male multiple personality. In each case the patient's mind, like my own, was filled with unique individuals having definite character traits. These personalities alternated in controlling the body and lived quite distinctive lives which the others often knew nothing about.

For example, as a multiple personality, my body was sometimes controlled by Linda, a violent woman filled with hate and capable of murder. At other times Charlene took over. She was long-suffering and capable of enduring great pain without complaint. Marie, another personality, was capable of loving others, being a mother, and working as a nurse. And so it went, each personality having a limited range of emotions quite different from the others.

Today I am Christina, a whole individual in my early thirties, with a normal range of emotions, whose life, though far from perfect, is totally within my control. Yet just a few months ago I was five years old—the same age I was when I disappeared into the "room" inside my mind to hide while my alter-personalities ruled my body for almost thirty years. How I disappeared and was "reborn" is the subject of this book.

To fully understand Linda and the forces that created her, it is best to go back to my childhood before she and the others were "born." Once my mind split, I was always a loner—the strange child nobody wanted to play with. The other children taunted me when I couldn't remember events that happened just a few minutes before. Even my brother and sister ridiculed me, making me the butt of their jokes or, in my brother's case, the partner of his lust.

I remember very little about the first couple of years of my life—years in which I was still myself, Christina. What memories I do have are of living in fear of my father whose troubled mind had crossed the line from extreme moodiness to insanity.

Most of my knowledge of my natural father is vague because my mother and grandmother were reluctant to talk about him. When he met my mother, he was a truck driver in California and was apparently quite popular and relaxed. He had an excellent sense of humor and my mother said he made friends easily with everyone they met during the early years of their marriage.

The first hint of mental difficulties came when he enlisted in the army prior to World War II. He was a short, muscular man who apparently rebelled at the discipline of the military. He became violent in the barracks, severely beating anyone he felt was not treating him properly. He was dishonorably discharged and spent the war years working as a longshoreman.

My brother Al was the first-born child, arriving in 1939, a year after my parents got married. He was adored by my father who played with him for hours on end. Both Al and my father had red hair, so they became known as "Red" and "Little Red." The two of them were inseparable.

Two years after Al's birth, my sister Miriam was born. The idea of a daughter delighted my father as much as he had enjoyed the birth of his son. He showered Miriam with attention, calling her his "little Rose." All his spare time was spent with the two babies and he seemed delighted when my mother became pregnant once more.

Around March of 1942, a couple of months before my birth, my father began changing radically. He started quarreling with my mother, picking fights for both real and imagined slights.

Soon my father was staying away from home for days at a time. He would pick up women in bars, spend the night with them, then beat them brutally if they displeased him. If my mother tried to reason with him when he returned home, she, too, would be beaten before he went storming back out into the night.

Finally my mother could take no more. She moved into my grandmother's house, taking Al and Miriam with her.

My father was furious. He went to Grandmother's house and terrorized everyone. He demanded that my mother return with him. She said that she'd only return if he changed his ways, something to which he agreed. They moved back together just a few days before I was born.

My birth was different from the births of my brother and sister. Perhaps having babies was no longer a novelty. Or perhaps my father's twisted mind no longer had room for children. Whatever his reasoning, he decided I wasn't worth his time or attention. He ignored me, leaving my care completely in Mother's hands.

My father's lack of love might have been easier to take had my mother been able to compensate for his coldness. But she didn't seem to care about me either. She fed me and kept me dry but ignored me the rest of the time. I can vividly remember being placed in a playpen in the sun where I would be left alone for hours at a time. Al and Miriam were frequently in the yard, but they were old enough to play quietly together. I longed for the touch and attention of people within my sight but always beyond my reach.

Having a third child made my father even more irresponsible than he had been before the separation. He began drinking heavily again. At first it was just in the evening, then earlier and earlier in the day until finally he was missing work altogether in order to "open" the bars. He went back to enjoying other women, but his spare time was primarily occupied with another self-indulgence—gambling. When the money ran out and we began missing meals, my mother bundled up the three of us and took us back to Grandmother's house.

My mother was pregnant during this period and the tension resulted in her giving birth earlier than expected. The premature infant, called "baby Art" by everyone, weighed just four pounds at birth. He had to be kept in the hospital until his weight increased another pound.

My father was notified of the birth of his second son and came over to my grandmother's house to see him as soon as the infant was released from the hospital. He forced his way inside, insisting the child needed a father's "loving" hand to be raised properly.

Father began tossing the infant up in the air, each time throwing him higher and higher. He called the baby a "runt" and a "sniveling bastard like his mother." And during this entire time, baby Art was being tossed into the air, caught, and tossed up again. It was as though Father was playing catch with the infant.

Grandmother was terrified. She told my father that he had seen his son and it was time to put him back to bed for his nap. Mother pleaded with him to stop. The pleading continued as Father kept tossing baby Art higher and higher.

Suddenly my father tired of his game. He balanced baby Art in his hand for a moment, then drew his arm back and hurled the infant against the floor. There was a loud, piercing scream followed by a wailing moan. The tiny body spasmed and then was still. Baby Art's nightmare had lasted but a few minutes; he lapsed into a coma, dying several days later.

My father was unmoved by the fact he had killed his son. He warned my mother that he would one day come for the three remaining children.

It was the end of November, 1944, when he made good his threat.

My mother opened the door for my father. She had learned that if he was truly determined to get inside, he would find a way.

My father looked at my mother for a moment, his body tense. His heavily muscled arm went back, then shot forward, smashing his fist into my mother's jaw. Her eyes glazed over as her body was propelled back across a chair. She was unconscious before she tumbled to the floor, her body a tangle of grotesquely twisted limbs.

We children were too small and frightened to offer any resistance. Father grabbed us and gave us some sort of drug he had brought with him. My next conscious moment found me in a pit squeezed against my sister. It was pitch black and we could barely twist our bodies. We didn't know if we were right side up or upside down. There were no sounds and no smells we could recognize. There was also no air. My head ached and I gasped for breath. I started to cry but that only used up what little oxygen remained. My chest became tight and I lost consciousness again.

For the next two years the three of us children barely existed. None of us has any memory of this time. It was as though we were in suspended animation. In my case, the only certainty is that my shoes were never taken from my feet. When we eventually left my father's control, it was found that my feet were mangled and crippled so badly that it was impossible for me to walk. My feet had tried to grow within the confines of the unyielding shoes and the result was an ugly mass of deformed bones.

Eventually my father grew tired of us. He decided to abandon us at an orphanage in Bakersfield, California. But first he had to commit the final outrage against me.

I have no memory of where it happened. Perhaps it was in a motel or even the car. All I remember is the act itself and that horror is as vivid in my mind as if it just occurred. It is something to which I may never fully adjust, even though my mind is no longer split into fragments from the experience.

My senses fixated on Father as he approached. First there was the smell—a strong odor of alcohol. Then came the sounds—an incoherent blend of muttered curses. I watched him as he came ever closer, his movements jerky and threatening. I pressed back against something—a bed, a wall, a chair—something that restricted my movement. I wanted to turn and run but my father blocked the only escape path.

Then there was the zipper. He pulled it down and reached into his pants, withdrawing his penis. My stomach was churning and I heard myself crying and pleading. I didn't know what was going to happen but I knew it was wrong.

Father slapped me. Once...Twice...Back and forth across the face while he stroked his penis erect. I stopped crying but the terror overwhelmed me.

I've done something wrong, I thought. I've done something terrible and now I'm going to be punished. But I don't know what I've done. I'm sorry, Daddy. Don't hurt me anymore. I won't do it again. I won't...I won't...

He reached for me, grabbing my panties and ripping them down. He held me so I couldn't move, his large hand clutching my neck and the upper part of my chest, his other hand guiding his penis toward my body.

There was a scream somewhere in the distance. At first it seemed to be coming from my throat. I felt the vibrations of my vocal cords and the rising pitch of sound emerging from my lips. I twisted my body but to no avail. The sound grew louder and louder as the penis was pushed against me.

Then there was the pain. The searing flash as the penis was thrust into my body's tiny opening, stretching and tearing the skin. The scream I was hearing rose to a painful wail, blocking all other sounds, then faded into silence. The person who had made the sound—me, Christina—was gone. My body was unable to physically flee the attack, so my mind handled the escape for me. At that moment I had made a mental leap into the nightmare world of insanity. I had become a multiple personality.

Marie awakened for the first time on a strange bed in a large room filled with countless other beds. She was thirsty, scared, and alone. Nothing was familiar.

How did I get here? thought Marie. She remembered something about Daddy and being afraid. There was the sound of a car and a sense of motion. She remembered huddling with Miriam and Al, but that was all. Even worse, their memories were no better than hers. Neither she nor they could make any sense of what had happened. Even in the orphanage the only security they felt came from knowing that the three of them were still together.

Why doesn't Mommy come for us? How can she let us stay here like this? Is Daddy coming back? There were so many questions and so few answers that made any sense to so small a child.

I've got to find somebody, thought Marie, swinging her legs over the side of the bed. She lowered herself to the floor. Her legs buckled and she toppled forward.

Marie reached for the side of the bed, pulling herself upright. This time she managed to balance her body on her shaking legs. Her feet ached, feeling twisted and cramped in her tiny shoes. She took a tentative step, one hand touching the mattress for support. Again her knees buckled and she fell against the side of the bed.

Suddenly the door at the end of the room burst open and several nuns came rushing to comfort Marie. Their clothing was unfamiliar to her but their words were gentle and their hands soothing.

The nuns explained to Marie that she was in the girls' wing of an orphanage and the room was empty because the other girls, including Miriam, were outside playing. Al was also in the orphanage but he was in the boys' section down the hall.

The nuns asked Marie her name and where she lived. None of the children could give them any information. It was obvious the children would have to be treated the same way as those whose parents were known dead. There seemed no way to ever reunite us with our mother.

Marie wet her bed the first night she slept at the orphanage and the nuns assumed it was an accident due to her emotional turmoil. They placed a rubber sheet on the bed and thought nothing more about it that day. The truth of the matter was that, until I was fourteen, I would be unable to go through the night without wetting my bed, but they didn't know this at the time. It was a few days before they realized I had a problem, and they decided to take drastic measures to "cure" me.

"You're a big girl, Christina," one nun told me. "You're five and a half, according to your sister, and that's too old to be wetting the bed. All the other children your age don't wet the bed so it's obvious you're doing it deliberately and we can't have that!"

The nun's words confused Marie. The name Christina

was a familiar one but she knew it wasn't hers.

If I'm not Christina, who am I? wondered Marie. She thought long and hard, though without success. She realized no one had ever called her by any name other than Christina, so it was up to her to name herself. The name Marie had a pleasant sound to it, though she did not realize that Christina Marie was my first and middle name before my mind fragmented during the rape. She thus adopted Marie as her own name, a name she would use for almost thirty years.

Marie wasn't worried when the nuns scolded her for wetting the bed. She couldn't help herself and thought they would understand. They had been so kind when she first awakened, she knew they would be gentle about this as well. She was mistaken.

One morning, a few days after her arrival, one of the nuns took the urine-soaked sheet from the bed, then wrapped it round and round Marie's face, pressing the wetness against her mouth. Only her nose was clear for breathing and her nostrils filled with the odor of her waste. Marie became nauseous but somehow managed to keep from vomiting. She knew that if she threw up, she could choke under the sheet.

I've got to stay calm, Marie told herself. Her heart was racing and she found herself gasping. Tears came to her eyes, but crying only made her breathe harder and that meant taking in more of the noxious fumes. Her nose filled with mucus and the thick liquid drained into her throat as she tried to pull air through her partially clogged nostrils. Her fear increased and she wanted to scream with terror. She began choking and coughing, then lost consciousness.

I can endure, thought Charlene. She managed to calm the cough reflex and bring the body under control. Marie had been overcome by fear but Charlene could handle the pain and terror which overwhelmed the others. Charlene was created to deal with pain. Charlene could experience anything the nuns chose to do to her without panic. She could ignore the odor of her urine and breathe comfortably despite the thick folds of sheet. Charlene was going to show the world she was a survivor.

Finally the sheet was unwrapped from Charlene's face and she could breathe normally again. I should go back into the mind, thought Charlene. I'm not needed anymore. She started to yield control of the body, then realized today's punishment was going to be repeated. She recognized that neither she nor any of the other personalities had control over the bed wetting. It would undoubtedly occur again that night and there would be more punishment the next day. There was a chance it would be even more severe, and neither Marie nor Linda would be able to cope. Charlene decided to stay in control for however long she was to be kept in the orphanage.

Of all my alter-personalities, Charlene was the most knowledgeable. She not only knew of the existence of Linda and Marie, she also knew everything they did or experienced. She knew that if they suffered pain or were put in danger, it was her job to rescue the body. Later, when Linda tried to commit suicide, it was Charlene who made certain I survived.

The nuns found the bed wet the following morning and, as Charlene expected, the punishment was intensified. One of the nuns decided that the nightly accidents were occurring because Charlene didn't go to the bathroom enough. She was ordered to sit on the toilet, relieve herself completely, and not get off until she was told she could.

And so Charlene began the nightmare that was with her day after day. Immediately after breakfast she would be ordered to the toilet, then forced to stay on the seat as the seconds became minutes and the minutes stretched into hours. Sometimes she would have the additional punishment of the wet sheet wrapped around her mouth.

I will endure, thought Charlene. I will sit here and endure whatever they require of me.

Charlene's legs began to ache. The muscles seemed to be cramping and she developed sores on her rear. When she was allowed to step off the toilet, the muscles felt as though they would double into knots, twisting her legs like a tightly coiled rubber band.

"You've got to learn to stop wetting the bed, Christina," the nuns told Charlene. They continued to use that name— the name that belonged to the "other" little girl who was too frightened to come out. It was upsetting not to be recognized for the individual she was, but Charlene felt this was the least of her problems. The physical abuse, though well intended, caused her body to feel as though it had been jabbed with hot pokers. A beating could not have caused her more discomfort than the endless hours on the hard toilet seat.

The bed wetting continued while the nuns became increasingly frustrated with what was happening. Not only were their punishments not working, they were being endured with stoic acceptance and a calm unnatural for a child Christina's age. There was no crying, no pleas for them to stop the punishment nor promises to be good. She just did what she was told, showing no reaction to either their abuse or their occasional affection.

Charlene lacked for companionship during this period, a fact which didn't bother her even though both Linda and Marie would have been upset without playmates. The other children banded together against the "baby" in their midst. They would taunt her for wetting the bed and upsetting the nuns. Only Miriam would play with her upon occasion, though Miriam preferred the company of the older children.

The officials at the orphanage decided they would have to keep me until I reached adulthood. I wet my bed and had feet so crippled I couldn't walk. They assumed my physical disability was permanent, and there were so many healthy, normal children available for adoption, it was doubtful anyone would want me. Only Miriam and Al were considered adoptable and they were placed fairly easily.

Al and Miriam were frightened by the change. They spent most of their time in the new home crying over the loss of their sister. Finally the couple who adopted them were so moved by their anguish that they agreed to adopt me, too.

Charlene remained in control of the body during the first few days in the new home. But the people were kind and Charlene could tell we weren't in any danger. She felt safe returning to her "room" in the boarding house of my fragmented mind.

Marie found herself sitting on a large, overstuffed chair in the living room of the ranch house. The room reminded her of someone's home but she knew it wasn't her home.

Grandmother? thought Marie. This isn't Grandmother's house. But it wasn't the orphanage, either. That building had much bigger rooms, with row after row of beds.

Marie was concerned, but she wasn't frightened. This was different from when she had awakened in a strange bed.

There were smells in the room, too. Someone was cooking her favorite foods. She got off the chair and followed the aroma until she found the kitchen. Al and Miriam were gathered about a table in one corner of the room, talking with a woman in her early forties. They glanced at Marie when she crawled into the room, but no one seemed surprised to see her.

Something was wrong. Marie realized that part of her life had disappeared from her memory. She didn't know what was happening or why the knowledge scared her. Everyone else seemed to understand where they were and why, but not her.

Gradually Marie came to understand her circumstances.

She discovered she was living on a ranch where Black Angus cattle were raised. She had been adopted by the couple who owned the place, as had Al and Miriam.

Marie understood, yet she didn't understand. Life seemed overwhelming for her and she wondered if maybe she was sick. Al and Miriam chatted happily about the events of the past few weeks, events Marie knew nothing about even though the others claimed she had participated in many of them. She tried to ask questions, but Al and Miriam were annoyed that she didn't remember as they did. They became so angry and disgusted with her ignorance that they refused to talk with her.

I've got to pretend I remember things, thought Marie. I've got to make believe I know what happened so Al and Miriam will play with me. I'm different than they are. I don't always know what happened yesterday or the day before. Maybe I'm a dummy like they say. But they won't play with a dummy, so I've got to pretend I'm smart like them.

Marie made the decision to adopt an approach to life she was to use until she successfully underwent treatment with Dr. Brewster. She became a liar whose skills would grow increasingly sophisticated in the years ahead. She would hide her ignorance of what happened during days and weeks of her life from those around her. She would pretend there was nothing abnormal about her widely varying behavior.

Marie also developed her memory to the point where she could remember even casual conversations many months after they occurred. She felt there was so much she couldn't remember experiencing, what she could recall she intended to remember exactly as it happened.

At first Marie accepted the idea that she was mentally a "dummy" because it was the only concept which made sense to a five-year-old. Later, when she was older and in school, she realized she could compete with the "bright" kids, and then she began to think her problem was more serious. She learned about mental illness and gradually came to the conclusion that she might be going crazy. But that fear was several years away. For the moment she accepted her brother's and sister's taunt of "dummy" because she had no other explanation. All she could do was lie about things she couldn't remember, hoping no one would spot her deceptions.

Of all the people Marie had known in her short life, the couple who adopted her were among the nicest. Not only did they care about the children, they also provided them with enough food to eat. Every night their plates were piled high with meat, vegetables, and other good foods in quantities they had previously seen only in stores.

The FBI learned where we children were living only after full adoption proceedings had taken place. A report was sent to my mother regarding the couple who adopted us, and she agonized over the question of whether or not to let us stay. The material advantages for us were enormous. Mother realized it would always be a struggle for her to put enough food on the table. The couple could provide us with a good education and plently of affection. But in the end, my mother decided she would rather have us at home, regardless of what that meant.

The trip back was uneventful. Marie was somewhat apprehensive about going home with Miriam and Al, but she didn't discuss her feelings with them. She had a vague memory of the women she was going to see and the place she was going to live. But in a sense it wasn't really her home or family. She had been "born" only after the kidnapping and this would be her first visit to the place where Christina had been raised.

When everyone arrived at my grandmother's house, Marie recognized it immediately. There was the slender walk leading to the house, surrounded on all sides by trees, thick green grass, and multicolored flowers in bloom. In the midst of the shade trees was a long, cushioned swing covered by an overhanging canopy.

"Frances, they're here!" shouted my grandmother. "Thank God, they're here!" She was standing on the porch, grinning broadly as my brother and sister ran up the walk.

One of the FBI agents opened the door for us, and Miriam and Al raced toward the house. Although Marie had started walking at the ranch, she had to be carried. She could only take a few short steps before having to quit, much like an infant. The couple who adopted us realized she wasn't a cripple when she was able to take those steps, but she had not learned to go any distance. Her damaged feet and long-unused muscles ached with each step and the pain quickly became unbearable. It would be several more weeks before she could walk reasonably normally.

A moment later Mother came to the door. Her face was soft and her eyes filled with tears of happiness. She grabbed Al and Miriam, taking one in each arm as the FBI agent carried Marie into the living room and set her on Grandmother's overstuffed green couch.

At first both Grandmother and my mother fussed over my brother and sister. But Grandmother quickly stood up and came over to see Marie. She hugged her tightly, kissing her forehead. Then she gently caressed her hair, saying, "Welcome home, Christina baby. Welcome home!"

But I wasn't home. At least I wasn't aware that I was. I was buried deep in the recesses of my mind.

2

DADDY BEN AND POVERTY –THE EARLY YEARS

Sometimes I am not certain whether my experiences with men were the result of bad luck or some sort of sick cosmic joke. My father raped me, my brother engaged in sexual deviation with one of my alter-personalities, husbands and lovers abused me. In fact, I have gotten to know only two truly kind men quite well in my life. One was Dr. Brewster, to whom I owe my restoration as a whole, mentally sound individual. The other was my first stepfather. The latter man started dating my mother shortly after the family was reunited following the ordeal of the kidnapping. I was no longer in control of my body then, but for some reason everyone accepted the strange behavior of my three most active alter-personalities.

My stepfather's name was Ben Watkins and he was adored by Marie and the other personalities. He was an unusual man—six feet six inches tall and extremely thin. He had been a professional baseball player but never got past the minor leagues. When he realized his athletic career would never provide much of a future, he became an entertainer. He had a rich, melodic voice and could play the piano more beautifully than anyone I had ever heard.

Daddy Ben, as we kids called him, was never destined for success as an entertainer, though. His jobs were in small clubs where people only half-listened while concentrating on their food, their drinks, or the small talk that might lead them to "score" with their date for the evening. Yet Daddy Ben loved what he did and preferred to be a low-paid traveling piano player rather than taking a better paying job outside the entertainment field.

Daddy Ben gave Marie the attention she had always lacked from her mother. The first day he came by Grandmother's house to meet us, he asked Marie if she would like to hear him play. Grandmother had an upright piano in her living room which she always kept in perfect tune. She, too, could sing and had taken lessons for several years. She used the piano every day to practice scales and other vocal exercises.

Marie was delighted to hear Daddy Ben play. She sat transfixed as his hands moved deftly over the keys. Sometimes the music was light classical. Other times he played the latest popular songs. Occasionally Grandmother would accompany him on the violin or they would sing duets. Al and Miriam became bored with such activity and went outside to play. But Marie was thrilled by every moment of it and demanded a concert every chance she got. Daddy Ben always complied.

Father was on the run during this period. There was a warrant for his arrest for the kidnapping of the three of us children as well as felony charges for armed robbery and other serious crimes. He had turned to a life of violence which caused my mother to live in constant fear. She prayed he would be caught before he could return and do further harm to the family.

My mother was in the process of getting a divorce during this period. Because of all that had happened, it wasn't necessary for her to locate my father to work out an agreement. She had become serious about Daddy Ben and just wanted to make a break with her past life.

Grandmother's house has become Marie's house. It was the one place she felt safe and loved. The living room had a big, overstuffed couch covered in a thick green fabric which doubled as the bed for we three children. There were also two chairs, one gold and the other dark brown, as well as an ottoman. A Persian rug, intricately woven, covered the floor. The piano and a music stand rested in one corner of the room and a small clock, like a miniature grandfather's clock, was on the wall. The small opening in back of the clock, meant to give access to the mechanism, was used by Grandmother as a "bank" for her emergency household money.

The kitchen was Marie's favorite room in the house. The floor was covered with linoleum that was so worn there were numerous holes in need of repair. The holes were covered by throw rugs which showed only slightly less damage than the floor. Grandmother never had enough money to make even patchwork repairs, though I never thought of her as being poor. The ancient refrigerator always held orange juice for us kids and she regularly baked us special treats.

When the divorce came through, Mother married Daddy Ben and the two of them rented the house next door to Grandmother's. We continued sleeping at Grand-mother's, probably to provide Mother and Daddy Ben with privacy, but our days were spent going back and forth between the homes.

Daddy Ben's deep love for my mother was obvious. Whenever he left town to spend a week or two playing in a distant club, he would take the time to write her lengthy love letters every day. When he was home, he treated us kids as though we were his natural children. He entered into our games and, in Marie's case, acted as confidant and friend.

It was during the time when we were still living next to Grandmother that Linda became active for the first time. Linda was first created during the rape. A part of my mind was outraged by my father's abuse. It wanted to lash out and hurt him—to break the fingers that held my throat and slash the penis penetrating my body. It was the part of me who, in later years, would be capable of killing without emotion. She despised Daddy Ben, not because she felt in any way threatened by him but rather because of the way he treated Marie. Linda wanted Marie to suffer. She didn't like the idea of Marie being happy and relaxed. If there was any way she could make Marie miserable, she would do it, no matter what might be involved.

Take the incident with the kittens, for example. Our neighborhood had a stray cat which was cared for by various homeowners.

The cat became pregnant and gave birth on the porch of the house in which Mother and Daddy Ben were living. Marie was fascinated by the kittens and immediately fell in love with them. She fondled them as though they were tiny babies. My parents were too poor to provide her with many toys and the kittens were a diversion more delightful than anything she had ever experienced.

So she likes those stupid kittens, thought Linda. I wonder what she'd do if she found them all cold and stiff, like little furry ice cream bars?

Linda picked up one of the kittens, carried it into the kitchen, and placed it in the freezer compartment of the refrigerator, closing the door when the animal was inside.

Linda left the refrigerator, got another kitten, and returned to the kitchen. She opened the door to put it inside, hoping the first kitten would be dead. It wasn't. It was barely moving and probably badly hurt, but it lived. The same was true for the second kitten and the third.

Marie was unaware of what happened to the kittens when she again had control of the body. They were the first she had ever been around during their early growing stages and she had no idea that the animals were being abused. They were having trouble moving about and were obviously sick, but Marie did not know enough about them to be aware of all this.

Linda began repeating her experimentation with the freezer every few days as the kittens grew larger. She figured that the more space they took up, the harder it would be for them to live. Yet they still managed to survive her abuse.

Finally Linda had had enough. Worthless little shits, she thought to herself as she looked at the tiny creatures. The kind of life you've been living, you're better off dead.

Linda walked over to the sink on the porch. She plugged the basin drain, filled it with water, then took the kittens, one by one, and forced their heads under the water. They clawed and fought her, but she didn't react. Deep scratches were gouged in her arms. Blood began flowing freely, coloring the water. But Linda did not relax her grip nor show any sign that she felt the pain. She held the kittens until every last breath of air had passed from their bodies and their lungs were filled with liquid. When she was done, every one of the kittens was dead. Then she took them out in the yard where the sun would dry the fur on their bodies and someone would be certain to find them.

There was a scream—low at first, then rising higher and higher in pitch until it was a shriek, echoing from the walls of the houses and carrying through the neighborhood. Several people burst from their homes to see what had happened. Marie was kneeling on the ground, a low moan coming from her throat, cuddling first one tiny corpse and then the next.

Marie finally got enough control to recognize that the dead must be buried. She found a shovel and held a funeral, praying intensely for the little kittens. Her arms stung where the sores had become infected, but she paid no attention to the pain. She had no idea how she came to have so many cuts and it didn't matter to her. Her injuries would heal. The kittens were dead and that could never be undone.

As Marie finished patting the last bit of dirt on the mound that served as a grave, she heard something far in the back of her mind. Even while she was crying steadily, there was the sound of laughter inside her head. It was distant and yet just below the surface of her brain. It was Linda mocking Marie from her "room" inside my mind.

In the years ahead, Marie would occasionally hear sounds in her head, including the voice of someone talking. She never quite understood the words and she never admitted what was happening for fear others would think she was crazy. She personally believed she was losing her mind and was terrified that she might get locked away forever. It was better to keep her madness to herself than to admit that something very wrong was occurring deep within her brain.

The period of relative stability that the family experienced during this time was shattered by a telephone call from my father. He had learned about my mother's marriage to Daddy Ben and wanted to destroy it. He talked about coming to the house to do physical harm to them and to us kids.

My mother decided that she and Daddy Ben had to take us and flee the city.

My family was always poor but we children never really felt the effects of poverty until we were traveling on the road with Daddy Ben. Then we began to eat cheap meals which never quite satisfied our appetites. Occasionally we had to go without food, a fact which the family accepted without complaint.

Marie, Al, and Miriam never begged for toys and presents. They would go into town, look in the store windows and long for the goods they saw, yet never mention their wishes.

Poverty bred ingenuity, and the three children soon developed games which could substitute for money. One of the games was "shopping" and it was played in the alleys behind the houses in the low-rent, slumlike neighborhoods in which we always lived. At least once a week, Al, Miriam, and Marie would go from trash can to trash can to see what had been discarded. A ripped dress, a ragged old hat, and some broken high-heeled shoes could transform Marie into a "queen." Dolls were loved even though they were missing arms, legs, and/or eyes. Games with parts and pieces missing were combined and new rules created to accommodate whatever was left. Mirrors with jagged edges, combs with missing teeth, and brushes suffering from partial baldness found their way into our home so Marie and Miriam could transform themselves into "great ladies." And pop bottles, the ultimate treasure, were converted into money at the rate of a penny apiece. Al used to use the money to buy an occasional model airplane he could assemble.

Just as Marie and the other children found a solution for the toy shortage, so they also resolved their hunger. Even when the family was extremely poor, my mother always tried to give us the treat of going to the movies. If she could scrape up a nickel each, she would send us to the Saturday children's show.

I'm hungry, thought Marie as she sat with Al and Miriam in the movie theater. Her stomach was churning and she could feel the intense pangs that occur when the body is denied what it needs for survival. All around her the other children were eating candy, cookies, and other treats.

Marie dropped to her knees and began crawling along the vacant aisles. First she'd locate an empty box. Then she'd fill it with the popcorn and candy the other kids had dropped or thrown during the show. Sometimes there would be a half-eaten sucker, other times a partial box of chocolate-covered raisins. It didn't matter what she found or what its condition. It was food and Marie was hungry.

The first real home Marie ever knew after all the

traveling was a nightmare structure we kids hated. We nicknamed the house "Ghastly Gables."

Ghastly Gables belonged to a grotesquely obese woman named Freda who had been a childhood friend of my mother's. Freda was about five feet two inches tall and weighed over 300 pounds.

Freda was married to a man only slightly less repulsive than herself. They had four children—two sons and two daughters—who seemed destined to be carbon copies of their parents.

Freda's family looked upon Ghastly Gables as a temporary residence when they lived there. They were saving their money and eventually built a larger home directly across the street. Since they felt themselves to be temporary residents of the Gables, they made no effort to keep the house clean. The stove was caked with dirt, grime, and food. There was moldly spaghetti sauce on the ceiling, and bits of graying pasta on the refrigerator. Cockroaches would scurry back and forth across the decaying food, luxuriating in the filth. Trash was stuffed into corners and the toilet was black, with an obnoxious odor no amount of flushing could end. The family lived like pigs in that horrible dwelling, then had the nerve to offer to rent it to my mother when they knew she and Daddy Ben needed a place to stay. To the horror of us children, my mother accepted the "generous" offer.

Mother didn't tolerate the filth, of course. Her first action was to clean the place so it was habitable. Disinfectant rid the toilet of its dank odor, but no amount of scrubbing could make the place attractive.

Ghastly Gables was set on a large corner lot, forty feet from the sidewalk. Grass was nonexistent but there was an abundance of dirt, pebbles, and yellow weeds. The cement walkway rose and fell at irregular angles. It was badly cracked, with weeds growing through every opening.

The house itself sat at an odd angle, as though there was

no foundation. Three steps led up to the entrance, each step creaking and groaning under the weight of even the smallest of us children. How Freda ever made it to the door without crashing through the steps is something I've always wanted to know.

The house had once been painted dark gray but it was peeling and partially bleached from the sun. Two windows faced the street, one of which was broken when we moved in and remained that way the entire time we lived there. Daddy Ben frequently talked about making repairs but he was only skilled with the piano. If he was ever lucky enough to select the right tool for the repair job he had in mind, he was usually not able to figure out what to do with it.

When you stepped through the front door, you found yourself in the tiny living room. A large, lumpy chair made even more unappealing by the roaches and other creatures living inside, and a worn couch with straw stuffing sticking through the holes were the main pieces of furniture. There was also a large lamp, the shade yellowed, mildewed, and torn.

As you passed through the living room, there was another room which held a battered double bed and a nightstand. Directly to the right was a closet just barely large enough to hold a cot. It was the "second" bedroom. Farther to the left was the bathroom where all the pipes were exposed. Rust stains permanently etched the sink, tub, and most of the plumbing.

Continuing through the house you came to the large kitchen. Olive green wooden cupboards lined the wall. Each had a door hanging from one hinge as though the effect had been planned by a deranged interior designer. There was a chrome dining room table and several chairs with torn seats and uneven legs.

The walls of the kitchen served as apartment housing for mice. The room was filled with the odor of damp mouse fur, an odor that no amount of cleaning could eliminate. Poison and traps were also of no use. The mice were just too firmly entrenched. In fact, I suspect that the mice were actually holding up the walls. The moment they left for new homes, the entire structure would probably collapse.

The electrical wiring was a fire department's nightmare. Sockets hung from overhead with adapters inserted so extension cords could be plugged into them. Wires were frayed and some were completely bare. Several worn electrical cords added to the illumination by sparking from time to time even when the objects to which they were attached were not in use.

The back porch had a defective, ancient ringer washer that apparently had a short circuit. As a result, the metal side always had an electrical current pulsing through it. If you touched the side while running the clothes through the wringer, you would get a bad shock. It was Miriam and Marie's job to wring out the clothing, and both were small enough that they inevitably felt one or more jolts as they reached up to operate the mechanism.

Behind the house was a garage that was so filthy and rundown it made the house seem like an elegant mansion by comparison. No one ever attempted to use it for anything, including storage. My brother Al, a fearless explorer who went everywhere else, never had the nerve to step inside. He knew he might not survive long enough to get back out.

There were several chicken coops in the back yard. They hadn't been used for years but no one took the trouble to clean them. The waste products of the long-gone birds stood in hard cakelike piles, sickening monuments to a most unpleasant existence.

The only nice thing about the property was a miniature orchard of fruit trees which produced a handful of fresh fruit every season. They might have supplied us with an abundance rather than a mere taste of fruit had anyone bothered to care for them. But they were neither fertilized nor pruned nor watered. If the winter wasn't too harsh and the summer wasn't too dry, they managed to survive.

Although neither the decrepit fruit trees surrounding Ghastly Gables nor the meager meals my parents could afford were adequate for our bodily needs, we discovered the surrounding land offered marvelous opportunities for easing our hunger. The area was partially a retirement community and most of the homes were loaded with fruit trees. There was also farmland nearby and several commercial orchards.

The living arrangements at Ghastly Gables were made even more complicated by its size. An aged, stained, and lumpy mattress was kept under the double bed in the bedroom. At night my parents would sleep on the double bed and Miriam and Al would sleep together on the mattress that had been pulled out from underneath. Marie's place was on the cot in the closet area. Marie wet my bed every night, so she was made the outcast. Although she knew Daddy Ben loved her and she understood that bed wetting was not conducive to good family relations, being banished to the closet area added further to Marie's feelings of rejection and isolation.

The sleeping arrangements had other ill effects. The constant closeness of opposite-sex children frequently leads to incest. And our family was not to be excluded from what some people consider the most obnoxious sexual abnormality of all, but that was a few years off.

While living at Ghastly Gables Marie developed ringworm.

Marie was horrified when she heard that her hair was to be shaved completely off. She was going through a period in life when she was keenly aware of her appearance and what others were thinking about her. The idea that she would lose all her hair seemed just another way to humiliate her. It seemed like further abuse from the mother from whom she needed so much affection—affection she felt was constantly denied her.

In a moment Marie was gone. Her heart, which had been racing as she became increasingly frightened about the future, was beating normally again. Her face became calm, serene. There were no more tears. She stopped pleading with Mother to leave her head alone. Charlene had taken control of my body and Charlene could cope with the disfigurement that was about to occur.

Mother was surprised by her daughter's sudden acceptance of what must be done, but she was too grateful for the quiet to question why her daughter suddenly submitted herself. Mother took Daddy Ben's razor and shaved the long strands of hair from Charlene's head. Then, using an ultraviolet light to spot stubble, she removed the remaining tiny hairs with a tweezer, plucking each one individually. The scalp became tender and the pluckings stung with increasing intensity. But Charlene said nothing. She neither winced nor cried. She endured.

Then Mother picked up a pot of hot Purex and slowly poured it over Charlene's head. The skin felt as if it was alive with fire. At first the stinging was on the surface. Then the skin seemed to crackle and split, breaking into a million tiny sores through which the hot Purex seeped down into the skull. Her brain felt like it was a pig being roasted on a spit.

The fumes from Purex were intense. Charlene held a towel tightly against her face to prevent the Purex from going into her eyes, but the fumes reached her nose and mouth, causing her to choke and gasp for breath.

Al and Miriam stood nearby, watching in awe. They were amazed by the inner strength "baby" Marie was showing. They knew they would have been crying and screaming with pain, yet their little sister was saying nothing.

The final humiliation came when Mother took some sort of turquoise-colored ointment and applied it to Charlene's head. The ointment seemed to glow, making her look a little like a warning beacon in the middle of a harbor. However, this was quickly covered by a white bonnet meant to prevent her from spreading the disease by touching something with her bare head.

When the ordeal was over, Charlene returned control of the body to Marie who was shocked to learn she couldn't remember the experience of having her head shaved. She stared into the mirror, looking at her bonnet and the traces of the turquoise ointment that remained visible. She wanted to rip off the covering and see exactly what had happened, but she didn't have the courage.

"We'll protect you, Marie," Al and Miriam told her. They said they wouldn't let the other children tease her. They would beat up anyone who made fun of the way she looked.

It was only when Al and Miriam promised to protect her that Marie realized there was another ordeal she had to face. She begged my mother to let her stay home from school until her hair grew out, but that was not permitted.

Daddy Ben, as usual, was able to offer the most support. The next morning he took Marie in his arms, hugged her, and told her he loved her despite what she was going through. He wanted to be certain she understood she wasn't being punished, that she really needed to have her head shaved in order to get well. "When this is all over, I'll make it up to you," he added. "I'll take you somewhere, just you and me. We'll spend a day together doing anything you want to do. Just remember that—we'll have a whole day together. I know some of the children are going to make fun of you in school. But don't you pay any attention to them. They're going to be cruel, but you do your best to ignore them. Promise me that, honey?"

"I promise, Daddy Ben," Marie said. And at that moment she meant it. Daddy Ben was the most wonderful man in the world to all my personalities and if he wanted Marie to endure something, no matter how humiliating, then she would make the effort.

Al and Miriam were fairly good about not teasing Marie. However, a cousin of ours came to visit with his mother one day. He took one look at Marie's bald head and promptly named her "Baldy Buzzard." For the next several years, whenever she had a fight with Al or Miriam, they taunted her with that name.

The worst part of the entire experience came many months later, after Marie's hair had grown back fairly well and she thought the long nightmare was over. The family had moved by then and Marie was going to school in Los Angeles. The kids didn't know her as a "freak" and everything was going smoothly. Unfortunately, the ringworm apparently came back, for the entire process of shaving, hot Purex, and ointment applications had to be repeated.

My childhood relations with Al and Miriam were as varied as the personalities who controlled my body. Linda was a violent fighter who liked nothing better than beating up one of the other kids or doing harm to what they held most precious.

For example, there was the time my brother Al made what he called "the Cadillac of Cadillacs." He was forever putting together pieces of junk of one sort or another. Usually he created "cars" which he would try to get Marie to drive. The "cars" invariably fell apart and caused great hilarity for those who weren't unfortunate enough to be in the driver's seat.

"The Cadillac of Cadillacs" was made from a wheelbarrow. An upside-down carton had been attached in such a way that it really did look like a small car. There was a windshield and a steering wheel, though none of the controls worked. It still had to be operated like a wheelbarrow.

Al proudly showed his latest invention to Marie and Miriam. He then announced he needed a driver, a statement Miriam ignored. She had no intention of getting inside.

"How come you need a driver when you can't steer it from the inside?" asked Marie. She never seemed to learn, from one experience to the next, that certain people would not change. Al's inventions were always going to be disasters.

"You've got to get inside, Marie," Al persisted. "I'll be steering it. Once you're inside, we can tear all over the neighborhood in it. I'll be your wheels; your engine. Come on, Marie. What do you say?"

Al had no intention of pushing Marie through the neighborhood, though. He was setting up a scheme for humiliating her as he had done so often in the past.

Marie climbed into the wheelbarrow as Al steadied it. From the outside it seemed like fun. Inside was another story. The wheelbarrow was some four feet above the ground and there were no hand grips. As Al lifted the back, Marie had to struggle to keep her balance. However, once he began pushing it, the ride didn't seem too bad.

The wheelbarrow picked up speed. Marie was on her knees, bent over and unable to see what was happening despite the hole Al had cut for the windshield. She was frightened by the gathering momentum. She pleaded with Al to stop but he made no response.

Suddenly the pushing sensation was gone. Al had released the wheelbarrow on a section of the street which sloped downward. The wheelbarrow was racing forward, skidding, bouncing, and moving crazily. Then it began to spin and Marie was thrown out. She tumbled and rolled, sliding along the pavement, cutting her face and her hands and tearing her clothing.

Marie grew dizzy. She stopped, put her hand to her

head, reeled slightly, then stood straight and defiant, a smile on her lips. There were no more tears.

Linda went back to the "Cadillac," bent down and picked up the broken pieces of wood and cardboard which formed the body of the vehicle. She set them in the wheel-barrow and pushed it back up the hill. Al and Miriam jeered at her as she passed, but she ignored their comments. Instead she pushed the wheelbarrow back to the house, out of sight of her sister and brother.

Linda parked the wheelbarrow, then walked to where Al kept his model airplanes. They were his most precious posses-sions. Each kit had been purchased with the money saved from selling empty pop bottles back to the stores at a penny each. It was always a long process to obtain and complete a model. First he would rummage through the trash cans looking for unbroken bottles. Then he would carefully hoard his pennies, depriving himself of candy and other immediate pleasures so he could save enough of the coins to buy a model kit and then the cement and paint needed to complete it. Finally he would painstakingly assemble the model plane, eventually placing his treasure on a shelf where he could admire it whenever he liked.

Linda picked up first one model and then the next. She carried them to the wheelbarrow, positioning the models among the pieces of wood and cardboard. Every model on the shelf was carefully arranged. Then Linda took a packet of matches, lit one, and set fire to the cardboard.

The flame was tiny at first. It spread slowly along the edge, gradually working toward the middle of the cardboard. The planes nearest the heat began to melt into blobs of colored plastic. Then the cement caught fire and the flames leaped explosively from plane to plane, melting and charring the plastic. Dark, acrid smoke rose from the wheelbarrow as Linda walked away. Even if Al spotted the smoke and was able to extinguish the fire, his precious planes would be gone.

Al had discovered the ruins of his airplanes. When you are as poor as we were, the few possessions any family member was able to accumulate took on greater importance than they might otherwise. Al wept unconsolably over the loss of his planes, and tears were still streaming from his eyes when Mother returned home.

"Marie destroyed your airplanes?" Mother exclaimed. "Well, I'll take care of her!"

Mother went to the closet, grabbed a heavy wooden coat hanger, and went looking for Marie. This third child of hers had always been a strange one. She insisted upon being called by other names and seemed to be different people at different times. But she had never been bad like this before. Destroying the models was just about the cruelest thing she could have done. Mother was going to see to it she never did anything like that again. When she finally found Marie, who unsuspectingly rushed happily toward her, she began beating her without mercy.

Marie, understanding what happened, accepted the punishment. She had learned that when someone accused her of something she couldn't remember, it was better to take the credit or the blame than to try and explain about not remembering. No one ever believed her and, sometimes, the explanation only resulted in more severe punishment.

Five miles from where Daddy Ben had rented a place for the family to live was a public swimming pool in which we children could play.

Usually Marie took the long walk to the swimming pool, the other personalities staying in their "rooms" while she enjoyed the water. But one day Linda decided to take control as Marie was walking to the public restroom at the pool. The switch was sudden, occurring as Marie walked past a woman sitting on a towel, an open purse resting on the ground at such an angle that the woman couldn't watch it.

Stupid, thought Linda. Dumb old bitch leaving her purse wide open like that. Anybody could take her money and she'd never know.

Linda walked over to the woman, making sure that not even her shadow crossed the woman's field of vision. She bent her legs slightly, dipping her hand in the purse and removing the wallet.

Linda remained in control of the body, saying nothing about her new wealth until the three children were returning home. Then she said, "Let's stop at the hot-dog stand." The stand was halfway to their home and they passed it every day, never being able to do more than wish for a taste of the food it sold. "We can buy as many hot dogs as we can eat!"

"And what are we supposed to use for money?" said Al. "Or are we so adorable they're going to just give the hot dogs to us?"

"Don't worry," said Linda, smiling. "I've got money." She stopped, pulled the money from her pockets, and showed it to the others.

The three children felt like royalty with so much money. They ordered chili dogs, Al eventually eating seven of them, Miriam and Linda consuming five each. They also devoured french fries and Cokes to complement the main dish of their "orgy." When they were done, only a few dollars remained. Linda stuck the money in her underwear and, when they returned home, hid it behind the flowered curtains in her bedroom.

When Linda submerged and let Marie return, Marie knew nothing about the money. It stayed hidden for several weeks until one day Marie happened to be staring out the window and saw the corners of the hidden bills.

Somebody must have left the money before we moved in, reasoned Marie. To her it was like a gift from heaven. She knew her parents wouldn't have used her room's window ledge to hide valuables, and Al and Miriam never had any money. This must be her own special gift and she wasn't going to share it with anyone. She grabbed the money, raced out the door, and ran to the dime store. She bought paperdoll books, coloring books, and crayons, happily carrying home her packages.

Daddy Ben and Mother were in the kitchen when Marie returned home with her bounty. Daddy Ben had been on the road for several days and was back home earlier than Marie had expected him.

"What have you got there?" asked Daddy Ben after hugging Marie hello.

"Some things I bought at the dime store," said Marie happily.

Daddy Ben's face grew serious. "Where did you get the money for all that?" he asked.

Marie suddenly realized something was wrong. Maybe the money wasn't a special gift from heaven. Maybe the money really belonged to someone else. If it did, and if she told the truth, she might be in real trouble with the man she adored. She decided she'd better lie about it.

"I got them with money I've been saving from collecting pop bottles. I found a lot of bottles yesterday behind a store."

"I don't believe her," said Mother.

"Give her a chance," said Daddy Ben. He and Mother had an agreement about raising the children. Although he showed us more love and affection than I ever felt from Mother, he agreed to let her handle all discipline. He was not to criticize what she said or did to us. However, he was going to make certain we got a fair hearing before any punishment was meted out. "Come on, Marie. I want you to take me where you say you found the bottles. It would take a whole lot of bottles to pay for all the things you bought."

Linda had been listening to the conversation from her "room" in the recesses of my mind. She was upset with the way the questioning was going. "I'm telling the truth," she shouted angrily. Her face was hard, her eyes intense. Adrenaline was rushing through her bloodstream and she was poised for a fight. She was ready to lash out at anyone, even Daddy Ben. "You two never believe me. I hate you both! I wish you'd go away and never come back!"

Daddy Ben had seen what he thought was Marie's fury at times in the past but this was the first time it had ever been directed against him. The intensity of her hostility upset him but he remained patient. Instead of angrily responding to the outburst, he quietly told Linda that he would like her to take him to the store where she claimed to have found the bottles. The two of them walked several blocks to a store where broken glass, garbage bins, and other debris were scattered around the back.

Daddy Ben studied the child in front of him. She was a paradox—at once hostile and frightened. He realized she had reason to fear her mother's type of discipline. Her treatment of her youngest child had been even harsher than her handling of Al and Miriam.

Finally Daddy Ben shrugged his shoulders and said, "I'm going to tell your mother I believe you, just to keep the peace. But I want you to know that I doubt you're telling the truth."

Linda learned her lesson from that experience—don't get caught. She stole frequently but she never again shared the money with Al and Miriam and she never bought anything she had to take home.

There were severe tensions within the family, tensions that left everyone fearful and uncertain about what tomorrow would bring. Mother and Daddy Ben constantly discussed my father, giving us the impression that at any moment he might force his way into our home and steal us away again. Mother seemed to feel Father had a special sense that would enable him to find us no matter how well hidden we made ourselves. She had to force herself to let us go outside, play, and lead normal lives, but she worried constantly and was near hysteria when we came home later than expected.

The living arrangements were oppressive. The only places Mother and Daddy Ben could afford were either so cramped that no one had any privacy or so run down they were ready for condemnation by the health inspector. The situation embarrassed Mother, who seemed to feel there was something bad about not having money. She was constantly on the defensive when talking with others, and her fears and frustrations helped keep everyone on edge.

Marie never felt the inner peace we assume is a part of childhood. She was pressured by hunger and by Mother's constant fear of Father's return. Moves were made with enough frequency that the only place that seemed like home was the house in which Grandmother lived. She felt no roots, no real sense of belonging to anything or anyone.

3

GROWING APART

Linda, who was in charge of my body through much of my childhood, was a cynic about the world in general and men in particular. She was the product of a rape and, with the exception of Daddy Ben, she seemed unable to find a male she could respect. Every relationship seemed to have a sick twist to it, even the one with her brother, Al.

I was nine years old when the incidents with Al began. Linda was in control of the body much of the time and she happened to be out when Al came home from school one day. He went over to Linda and Miriam who were playing together and said he had learned a new word.

"What is it?" asked Linda.

"Fuck," he said, proudly.

"What does that mean?"

Al explained as best he could, not fully understanding, as he had not yet reached puberty. He wanted to try it, though, and Miriam and Linda agreed. Miriam seemed to instinctively know it was wrong the first time she tried it but she didn't try to argue with her brother and sister when they decided to keep doing it. Miriam made it clear that she would not tell on them, though she wanted nothing more to do with the situation.

At first the relationship was nothing more than child's play. At no time was there any affection between brother and sister. Linda and Al never kissed or clung together. They just went out back, where the ancient chicken coops were rotting in the sun, took down their pants, and rubbed their genitals together. They both liked the feeling it gave them but they were too young to have full sexual experience. It was several months before Al had his first erection, though once he did, they graduated to regular intercourse.

Marie had no knowledge of Al and Linda's actions. She would have been sickened by the thought and was never approached by Al to have sex. He seemed to sense when Linda was present, for it was only with Linda that he tried to have intercourse. He knew that there were times when his sister didn't seem "in the mood" and he left her alone at those moments.

Al and Linda continued having sex for the next two years. They were never caught, though they did have a close call one day. It happened when Mother wasn't expected for at least an hour. Al asked Linda about having intercourse, something they hadn't done for several weeks. Although they didn't do it regularly, they did it with enough frequency so that it was often on Linda's mind. She was older and had come to a better understanding of her body than she had when they first started.

"I don't know if we should do it anymore," said Linda. "I've been hearing things about it. You can get me pregnant doing it. Did you know that? I don't want to go having a baby. Someone told me once that if a brother and sister have a baby together, the baby will be a monster. I mean a real monster, with a funny-looking head and all, and it will be crazy to boot!"

"Ahhh, those are just old wives' tales," said Al. "Come on. You like it; you know you do. Please?"

But Linda remained reluctant.

"Hey, I know what," said Al. "I promise that if you'll do it with me, I'll be your slave for a whole day. I promise I'll do whatever you tell me to do. You know, like a servant. How about it?"

Linda thought about the proposal. She liked the idea of

Al being her slave. She would enjoy running him ragged. The image of his doing anything she wanted delighted her. "Okay, but this is going to be the last time. I mean that!"

The two of them went into the chicken coop and removed their pants. Al had a full erection, for he had reached puberty by then. Linda got down on the floor and Al put his penis in her. There was no other touching.

Linda watched the ceiling, enjoying the sensation between her legs and otherwise remaining coldly detached. She watched a fly land on her brother's head, listened to the sounds of the distant street traffic, and the noise of the children at play in the yard of a home two or three houses distant. Al began pressing against her rhythmically, harder and harder until at last he was done. Then he got up, put his pants on, and looked out a small hole in the wall which faced the street bordering the back yard.

"Oh, no!" said Al. "God damn, it's Mom. She's home early from work. Hurry up and get your pants back on. I'll go up to the house. I think I can beat her to the door. You stay here and come in later. And don't get that stupid look on your face that you always get when you've done something wrong. Mom can spot that look a mile off. It's a dead giveaway."

"Okay," said Linda, annoyed. "Don't get so steamed up. I'll wait here. You don't have to worry about me. I know what to do."

Linda put on her jeans after Al left, then picked up a piece of straw from the floor of the coop. She chewed on it to pass the time. She had no thoughts about what she and Al had done. The act of intercourse had brought her some pleasure, yet she would take far greater delight in humiliating him later when he became her servant. After a few more minutes, she went into the house.

"What have you been up to?" asked Mother. She was sitting at the table, having a cup of coffee and talking with

Al. "No good, I suppose."

"Lay off, Mom," said Linda. "I was out playing in the persimmon tree in the back yard. It's been too hot to stay in the house and I can get a good breeze when I sit up in the branches."

Mother didn't say anything further to Linda. Al asked Mother about her day at the factory and she immediately returned to that subject. She delighted in talking with Al about her work, as he always pretended to be interested.

Mother and her precious Al! thought Linda as she left the room. If Mother knew he'd just finished putting his dick in me, I wonder what she'd do. Probably beat on me and just give him a lecture. Yeah, that's how it would work. I'd get the pain and she'd only talk to him. Well, screw her!

Linda used Al as her main model of what a male is like. Daddy Ben was something separate; something special. She never saw him in the role of husband or lover in her fantasies. Instead she imagined that all men in her life would be like Al or what little she remembered of the crude, violent nature of my real father.

The days with Daddy Ben quickly came to an end the same year Linda began experimenting sexually with Al. One night Daddy Ben was playing in a nightclub near our home. He returned to the house in the early hours of the morning to find my mother standing naked in the yard, tearing weeds from the ground.

"What are you doing?" asked Daddy Ben, horrified.

Mother said she was picking roses—beautiful roses. She was making herself a bouquet to wear to the ball.

Daddy Ben rushed Mother into the house, got some clothing on her, and took her to the emergency room of the hospital. She was placed in the psychiatric ward and later taken to a long-term care sanitarium where she stayed for the next year.

That next year was an unpleasant one for my alter-personalities. Miriam went to live with Grandmother and Marie was sent to live with my Aunt Lucille. Al was taken on the road by Daddy Ben, who felt he could handle Al's education despite the traveling. Marie was crushed.

Aunt Lucille's husband was a dentist who later went on to earn an M.D. degree as well so he could become a dermatologist. Both were social climbers who rarely visited my Grandmother or any relatives on our side of the family.

Their home was a three-bedroom, two-bath, split-level in the nicest part of town. The furniture was antique white and gold, and all of it carefully arranged. Aunt Lucille became irate when anything was out of place.

She had one child of her own, a daughter who was not quite three years old. The child was too young for Marie to play with, but Marie was keenly aware of the difference in Aunt Lucille's attitude toward the child. While her own daughter was given lavish attention, Marie was treated as another piece of furniture. Marie was fed, clothed, and sent to school, but there was no love nor any attempt to ease the pain of having a mother in the sanitarium.

My aunt enrolled Marie in the neighborhood elementary school. The other children in the school had known each other all their lives. They came from similar upper-income backgrounds and their experiences were far different from Marie's. They were cruel in the way children can be and treated Marie like an outcast. Often they made fun of her background.

Marie couldn't handle the pressures of the hostile kids at school. She tried to avoid being with them, frequently fleeing into the recesses of my mind and letting Linda take over.

Each day Aunt Lucille packed a lunch for Linda that was bigger and more nourishing than anything Linda had received from her parents. But Linda decided she should steal additional food. It wasn't a matter of being hungry. She just enjoyed the thought of some other child going hungry.

Usually Linda did her stealing during recess. Since the other kids played games among themselves, not wanting this stranger in their midst, Linda wasn't missed when she sneaked away. She went into the classroom area where the lunches were kept, then placed the lunch she selected under her sweater when no one was watching. Eventually she took the bag to the rest room and tore it open to see what "goodies" it held. Cupcakes, cookies, and other foods of special delight would be consumed at once. Anything she didn't want would be torn into small pieces and flushed down the toilet.

Linda didn't just steal lunches, though. She took pencils, erasers, crayons, and similar items from the desks of the other children so they would be lacking tools essential for doing their class work. When the teacher was out supervising the recess activity, Linda was often able to find coins in her desk which could be spent at a small store two blocks from the school. Usually she bought a bag of candy with the money, eating her fill, then taking the remainder back to the school yard. She would shout to the other kids, "Come on! Here's some candy!" Then she'd toss the unwrapped pieces into the air and let them fall to the ground where the other children would eagerly scoop them up.

Linda tried not to admit to herself that she craved affection and personal attention. Yet she wanted to feel special, to be "somebody" in the eyes of those around her. Perhaps it was the reason she slept with Al. Certainly it was why she felt compelled to steal from the children who rejected her. Daddy Ben was the only person who had ever made the effort to appreciate her and now he was gone as a result of her mother's mental breakdown.

Linda lived with her aunt and uncle for several months before Aunt Lucille arranged for me to visit Grandmother.

Linda became increasingly excited during the drive to Grandmother's house. Her feelings of joyous expectation mounted as she leaped from the car and ran along the narrow walkway leading to Grandmother's front door.

Linda listened to the sounds within—the laughing voices of both Grandmother and her sister Miriam, the rattling of the dishes as they prepared dinner, and all the other happy "noises" that were a part of the house she remembered so fondly. But this time Linda suddenly realized she was listening with the ears of an outsider.

They're not going to get me, thought Linda. They're not going to hurt me.

Grandmother was delighted to see Linda. She hugged her and, for the moment, everything was as it had always been. Grandmother wore a flowered-print nylon dress and perfume which smelled like fresh roses. She had "sensible" walking shoes and a clean handkerchief in her pocket. The latter was ever present for emergencies such as the runny noses of her grandchildren.

Grandmother was a small woman, not even five feet tall. When Linda hugged her, she could see over Grandmother's shoulder into the kitchen where Miriam was standing. Linda's face took on a shocked expression, then she burst into laughter. During the time the sisters had been separated, Miriam had gained at least seventy-five pounds.

Miriam burst into tears, ran toward the back bedroom, and slammed the door behind her. "The blimp can really move when she wants to," said Linda, her voice loud and harsh. "Is she going to let companies paint advertising messages on her side?"

Grandmother looked at Linda in surprise. "What on earth is wrong with you? Why should you hurt your sister's feelings so?" She left Linda standing in the kitchen while she hurried after Miriam to comfort her. It was not the reunion everyone had expected.

The visit to Grandmother strengthened Linda's cynical view of the world. There was no love to be had from anyone. People either used you, abused you, or abandoned you. The only person she could count on was herself.

4
ADOLESCENT MADNESS

The fragmented mind of a multiple personality seems to become more clearly defined with the passage of time. When my mind shattered during the rape by my father, the three "people" who were formed each had specific roles to fill in order to help me funtion in life. Yet none of them could be considered "whole" individuals at "birth." Their characters were shaped in large measure by their life experiences.

Linda, for example, became increasingly dominant as I entered into adolescence. This is a period when growing up is difficult under the best of circumstances. The normal pressures of school, the developing sex drive, insecurity about the future, uneasiness about social relationships, and all the other adolescent difficulties overwhelmed Marie. She coped the only way she knew, "running away" into my mind while the hostile, independent Linda took control.

One of the reasons Marie felt she couldn't cope with life very well was the loss of the only man she had ever truly adored. When I was ten years old, my mother was released from the sanitarium. Instead of returning to Daddy Ben as we children expected, she informed us she was divorcing him.

My mother wasn't the type of woman to live alone. She needed a man, both emotionally and financially. Without Daddy Ben's meager income, our situation became critical. Mother went to work early in the morning and did not return until late at night. We kids had to take care of ourselves, and once again we experienced the days of little more than catsup sandwiches for supper.

When weekends came, Mother went husband-hunting. Mother always stayed out late on Friday and Saturday nights. When we children arose, there was a trail we could follow to indicate how she had come home. The earrings were usually on the sink and her shoes were on the floor, kicked off at odd angles. The petticoats would be found farther into the house, left in a rumpled heap. The bracelets would be on the bathroom sink and, finally, Mother would be stretched out on her bed. She was invariably hung over from too much drinking.

No matter what my mother did to me, no matter how hostile my feelings remain toward her, I have to admit she was concerned about us at that time. She never brought one of her dates home with her for a casual affair. We never met any of the men in her life until she finally became serious about one.

The man's name was Jacob, and Marie liked him immediately. He was a rather nondescript individual, quiet and interested primarily in his work. He was a mink rancher and he owned a green Chevrolet pickup truck which he used for his work. He always brought it with him when he took our family on outings. We kids lived to climb into the back and get taken to Marine World and similar places. It was the first time we had ever been to amusement parks that required what, for us, was a high admission price.

Jacob and Mother apparently had decided to get married before we met him, and they were concerned about how we would like him. He filled us with hot dogs and popcorn and so many good times that we quickly adored him. When she said he was going to become our new father, we were all pleased with the thought. He wasn't as special to Marie as Daddy Ben had been, but he seemed to love all three children equally and that was special in itself.

The one period during which Marie managed to maintain primary control came when the family moved to Torrance, California, for the first year after the marriage. The new home was ten miles from where Grandmother lived and an area where Marie, for the first time in her life, made friends with the other children in school. She and Miriam were in junior high and were made to feel truly welcome by the other students. They didn't care about where Miriam and Marie came from, how much their parents made, or anything else. They were willing to get to know them as individuals, and many of the students liked what they saw. In a short time, Marie and Miriam were a part of the school's "elite."

Marie was becoming quite attractive and she received the attention of a number of boys. There was one special boy in Marie's life during this period. His name was Bill, a bright, reasonably good-looking, and quite popular youth who was totally taken with Marie.

Linda stayed suppressed during most of that year. Marie attended school regularly and got top grades in her classes. She began horseback riding and spent hours with friends. She was blissfully happy, the period of boundless joy seeming to ease the hurt of all the years of loneliness. There was so little pain or frustration that Linda's aggressive strength and total hostility simply had no place in my existence. It was thus the calmest period I had ever experienced as a multiple personality and would be the only serenity I would know until after Dr. Brewster made me whole once again.

At last Marie was certain her life was going to be lived the way she always dreamed. She wasn't close to her mother and stepfather, but she had plenty of friends and was constantly on the go. She had developed a sense of self-worth and felt life was wonderful.

"Your stepfather and I have something to tell you," Mother announced one evening. "You know how Jacob has been talking about mink ranching? We finally decided that if we were ever going to make the move to start our own business, now is the time. We just put a down payment on a mink ranch out in the country. I know it'll be hard to move but you'll grow to love the new place even more than you love this one."

She's done it again, thought Marie. I've seen her watch me when I'm with my friends. I've heard the comments she's made about how much happier I seem where we're living now than any time before. She knew how I felt about this place and deliberately decided to take my happiness from me. She doesn't care about a stupid mink ranch any more than the rest of us. She just encouraged Jacob because it's a way for her to hurt me.

Tears streamed down Marie's face. She ran from the room, not wanting to give her mother the satisfaction of seeing her cry. She had no idea what she would say to Bill and her other friends. She was certain she would never again know such happiness, and her fears proved correct.

The ranch was six and a half acres in size, just a few miles from Santa Cruz. At the time, Santa Cruz, the nearest "big city," was a small resort town catering to crowds of summer tourists. In winter almost no one lived in the community.

Santa Cruz itself sits on the California coast approximately seventy miles south of San Francisco. The town to which my parents moved us had fewer than 200 people, though it is now a bedroom community and student haven since the University of California opened a branch in Santa Cruz.

The farmland surrounding the ranch had been owned by the same families for many generations. A number of the farm owners were interrelated. All of the families were friends, since for generations they had grown up together in the same small area, studying with the same teachers. It had been many years since the school children had seen "outsiders" and they were hostile to Marie, Al, and Miriam. They neither wanted to get to know the new family nor wanted to include them in their activities.

How can they hate us so much? wondered Marie. We haven't done anything to hurt them. They say we're from the city and that city people aren't good. But how do they know?

Marie tried to talk with her parents about the problems she was facing in school. But Jacob was too busy to listen and Mother didn't care.

I think she's glad I'm having problems, thought Marie. I think she's glad I'm not happy. She's never wanted me. She's never liked me. I try to please her and she rewards me by bringing me out here where I'm miserable. I've got to get away, I just don't know where to go.

The ranch house, a high-ceilinged wood building with seven rooms, was painted white on the outside, with green trim, and sat on the top of an incline in the center of the acreage. The ranch cost $12,000 when purchased in 1952 and sold for $75,000 ten years later.

The interior of the house was knotty pine and the floors were made from redwood. There were three bedrooms, a large bathroom, an enormous living room, and a kitchen that was equal in size to the living room. The entire house was sprawling, yet the only way to heat it was with a single oil-burning stove which made so much noise when lit that Marie lived in terror of its exploding. Only my stepfather touched that oil burner, as everyone else was afraid to go near it.

The kitchen stove was run on butane, and the first person to awaken in the morning was expected to light it for whatever additional heat it would provide. Oil was so expensive that all heat was turned off at night, and the temperature could get down to ten degrees above zero in the wintertime. Each of our beds was piled high with blankets and we used to sleep wrapped up like mummies.

The ranch land had been cleared with the exception of the southern edge where the natural vegetation had been allowed to grow wild. There was a pump house on the grounds, a small pond, and berry bushes that were loaded with fruit in the summer. There were also seven different varieties of apple trees and the apples became a major part of our diet.

The mink were kept on the northern portion of the property. Sheds contained the rows of wire cages in which the animals were housed. There were 5,000 mink at the peak of the business. There was also a cow and a few other animals.

Each of us kids was required to work with the mink and that meant tasks which could be dirty, smelly, and physically quite taxing. This was especially true during the pelting season. Once a year the mink prime their coats; they are then killed, skinned, fleshed, and the skins are put on boards to dry before being sent to the tannery in New York. After that, they go to an auction house where manufacturers buy them for use in coats, stoles, etc.

Marie was surprised by the amount of work she and the others were expected to do. She had not been raised on a farm and was unfamiliar with the many chores involved with a business such as the mink ranch. She may have been miserable over the years, but at least she had always experienced personal freedom. Suddenly she was spending as many hours doing assigned chores as she was spending in school. She felt as though she was being punished for daring to enjoy the first year of Jacob and Mother's marriage.

To make matters worse, none of the kids was paid for his efforts on the ranch. They saved Jacob the cost of hired help but little of the profits were spent on the family. Instead he put what he earned right back into the business. We kids were given the necessities but no money for high school yearbooks, class rings, and other items that are so important to teenagers.

Mother took the penny-pinching to an extreme. When Miriam reached puberty, she developed breasts so large that they bounced noticeably when she walked. She asked my mother for money to buy a bra because the kids at school were teasing her. She would have used the money from the rabbits she was raising, but they were not yet old enough to be sold. She could barely afford the food the rabbits ate.

Mother must have understood how humiliating it was to have the other kids tease Miriam about her emerging woman-liness. But if she did, she certainly didn't show it. She said she had no money for such foolishness, a statement which shocked Marie.

Marie was basically honest. Linda's actions over the years were definitely not part of Marie's moral code. Her life had been one of virtue and decency, and she was totally unaware of how Linda used her body. But when Marie learned that Mother wouldn't buy Miriam a bra, she broke with her code.

Mother doesn't have to listen to the teasing. She doesn't have to watch the boys deliberately bumping into Miriam. She doesn't hear the dirty jokes or the voice of that creep who told her she should come to his father's dairy farm so he could milk her.

Marie didn't have any money but she decided she wouldn't let that fact stop her. She went to Woolworth's and nervously shoplifted a bra. She felt horrible, robbing a store for something her mother should have purchased. Yet she saw no alternative. Miriam couldn't wait until she saved the money herself.

Al and Marie worked in the feed room. There was a large electric grinder, a fifteen-foot-deep, walk-in refrigerator, and a two-ton mixer. The animals had to be fed fresh meat every day and the feed was specially ground. Since the ranch was independent, everything had to be done by the family.

Mother's job was driving the ranch truck. She traveled hundreds of miles a week to different sections of northern California where she picked up supplies. She left early in the morning and arrived home late in the afternoon, following a regular routine.

Marie hated the feed room because it seemed like a mad doctor's laboratory in some horror movie. She would always disappear as she approached the building. In her place was Linda who took ghoulish pleasure in grinding the rabbit heads, fish heads, tripe, beef liver, chicken heads, and similar "goodies" which were mixed with Purina Mink Chow, cottage cheese, eggs, and vitamin supplements. The mink usually ate better meals than our family.

Marie, who controlled the body outside the feed room, fell in love with the mink, even though they were vicious creatures with fangs sharper than those of a wolf. The mink were the only creatures, animal or human, that seemed to accept Marie's presence.

Although Marie loved the animals, they were a poor substitute for human companionship. She longed for a conversation with Mother and Jacob, but their lives revolved around the ranch and each other. Even Al and Miriam were ignored in favor of the new business venture. Yet Marie had so many questions to ask, so many problems she needed help in resolving. Her difficulties were overwhelming and she found herself increasingly having blackout spells in which the events of previous hours or days were not remembered.

As the days turned into weeks, at least one student had a change of heart concerning the "strangers" who had enrolled in their school. A boy named Walter became attracted to Marie. He gave her a feeling of belonging she couldn't get from anyone else. As a result, she clung desperately to him.

Marie had finished her chores and wanted to ride into town with Miriam. There were still a few hours before it was time to feed the mink and she was anxious for a diversion. Miriam refused to let her come, though.

Marie was upset. She saw no reason why she shouldn't be allowed to go along. She asked why she wasn't wanted but Miriam tried not to tell her. Finally Miriam admitted that she wasn't just going to buy groceries. She was also going to the drugstore where she was picking up some pictures she had taken a few weeks earlier.

Suddenly Marie remembered. A few of the pictures were of herself with Walter. He had no pictures of himself he could give her when she asked for one. Thus she had no tangible evidence of their relationship that she could look at when they were apart.

Miriam agreed to take Marie into town to get the photographs. Even better, she understood Miriam to mean that Marie could keep the prints as well.

Miriam drove the new, large Studebaker pickup truck Jacob owned into town while Marie sat in the passenger seat, happily smoking a cigarette. The sisters pulled up in front of the store and Marie sat in the pickup truck while Miriam did her shopping.

After what seemed like hours, Marie spotted Miriam coming from the drugstore. She was carrying the bags of groceries and undoubtedly had the photographs as well. Marie began waving at her frantically, urging her to come faster. "Hurry up! Hurry up!" she shouted, but Miriam merely frowned and continued at a pace Marie found agonizingly slow.

Miriam reached the truck, dropped the bags of groceries onto the rear bed of the vehicle, then climbed inside. She put the key in the ignition and started the truck.

"Hey!" yelled Marie. "Where do you think you're going. I want to see those pictures right now!" She reached over and turned off the ignition switch.

"Stop that!" said Miriam angrily. "We're going home. Get your hands off the steering wheel and let me start the truck." She turned the key switch again.

"Don't you understand . . . ? Don't you understand . . . ?" said Marie, attempting to put her feelings into words. "The pictures . . . Walter . . . You've got to stop. You've got to show them to me . . ." Her heart was racing. She was angry with her sister and the rage building inside her was impossible to handle. She wanted to yell, to explode, but all she could do was stammer vainly. As she struggled for the right words to say, her world seemed to go black.

"You promised me you'd let me see those pictures," said Linda, her voice coldly menacing. She wrenched Miriam's hand from the ignition, her fingers digging into her sister's flesh. With her other hand she took the key from the slot. "Now, God damn it, I'm going to see those pictures!"

Miram tried to argue.

Linda felt pure hate for Miriam and was going to have her way no matter what. "You bitch! You God damn bitch!" said Linda. She slapped Miriam across the face, her open-handed blow having the impact of a boxer's fist. Miriam's head jerked to the side, slamming against the window of the truck.

Linda glanced around the parking area and saw it was empty. She opened her door, holding the ignition key in her hand, leaped out, and went around to the driver's side. She opened the door, then grabbed the astonished Miriam's pony-tail, jerking it hard and forcing her sister to the pavement. Her shoulder seemed to crack as it hit the hard ground.

"You're trying to play tricks with me again," said Linda coldly. Miriam was lying on the ground, holding her aching shoulder. "It's just like when we were little and you and Al used to gang up on Marie and make an ass of her. You used to laugh at her and you'd laugh at me when I took control. But that's over now. You're nothing but a fat, ugly pig and I'm going to knock the shit out of you. You're going to feel the pain you've been making me feel all my life. You're going to cry and plead and wish you had never, ever done anything to hurt me."

Miriam couldn't comprehend why her sister was referring to "Marie" as though talking of someone else. But before she could reply, Linda began striking her face. The blows came slowly at first, then increasingly rapidly.

Linda grabbed Miriam's shoulders and pushed her down,

striking her head against the concrete. Miriam lay on her back, blood flowing from her nose and mouth.

Linda jumped on top of her sister and ripped at her blouse. Then she rolled her sister over and completely removed it. Miriam was no longer able to resist. Her breathing was shallow and she was barely conscious.

Linda rose to her feet, looked down at her victim, and said, "God damn fat, ugly pig." Then she kicked Miriam hard in the stomach, climbed into the truck, and let out a deep sigh. When she attacked her sister, she did something she had wanted to do for several years. The violent act proved a great relief for her. At the same time, she realized there was a chance that she had killed Miriam. Her sister hadn't reacted to the kick in any way. Her body was lying on the ground, naked above the waist, with blood flowing from her head. She made no sound nor any attempt to move.

If Miriam's dead, I'm in trouble, thought Linda. I've got to get out of here. Quickly she receded into my mind.

What am I doing in the driver's seat? thought Marie. And where's Miriam? She was just in the truck a moment ago. We were . . . We were arguing and then I felt funny and . . .

Marie looked down at her hands. Her knuckles were raw and bleeding. Her clothing was dirty. Something had happened but she had no idea what. "Miriam?" she called through the window, looking all about for her sister. "Miriam?"

But there was no Miriam in sight. Marie became frightened, then glanced at the ground. Miriam was on her back, injured. For a moment she thought they had been attacked by a mugger who had hit her on the head. That would account for her not remembering the violence.

But it wasn't a mugger who had beaten Miriam, and somehow Marie realized that. It was her responsibility. She tried to remember what had happened during the last few minutes but she had no memory. She had one of her blackout spells and this time something really serious happened. Fear overwhelmed her. She started the ignition and floored the accelerator.

Marie headed along the road to the ranch, not knowing where else to go. Driving eased some of her tension and she realized she should have gotten out of the cab to see if she could help her sister. She knew she hadn't been thinking clearly when she drove away.

As Marie drove, she saw Gary Farleigh, a friend.

She explained that Miriam was in trouble and needed his help. Gary agreed to take the truck, leaving Marie standing by the road. She walked off to the side, into some high grass where there were a number of small pine trees she could hide behind. She stayed where she could see every vehicle coming along the road without the people in the passing cars and trucks being able to spot her.

After what seemed like an endless period of time, Marie spotted the Studebaker bouncing down the road. She saw two heads sitting up on the seat and knew Miriam was all right. As the truck passed, she saw that Miriam was holding her bloodied head in her hands. But at least she was alive! Whatever Marie had done during the blackout couldn't have been as serious as it looked at first.

Marie began walking slowly toward home. As she walked, she tried to think what might have happened. She remembered the frustration she felt about the photographs and how angry she had started to become. But when she attempted to express her rage . . . When she attempted to express her rage . . . That was the problem.

Al, Mother, and my stepfather were sitting at the yellow wooden table when Marie walked through the kitchen door. She felt very small and frightened. She looked around for Miriam but her sister was nowhere in sight.

Mother became enraged when she saw Marie. Her face was red and her fists clenched tightly together as she rose from her chair, shouting. "You little bitch! You God damned snot-nosed little bitch. You're as bad as your father. You almost killed your sister and now you've got the nerve to come walking through that door like nothing happened! I'm going to get the biggest damned board I can find and batter every inch of your skin until it will be a miracle if you ever walk again."

Jacob was startled by his wife's response. He was angry about what happened to Miriam but he thought my mother wasn't handling her temper as well as she should. "Now take it easy," he said to Mother. "Don't get so riled. Let's hear Marie's side of all this before you go off half-cocked." His voice was calm. He was concerned, but he was basically a man who saw no sense in punishing violence with violence if it wasn't necessary.

"Keep your nose out of this!" yelled Mother. "They're my kids. I told you when we got married that I'd make all the decisions involving them. They're my kids and you're not to tell me what to do or how to do it. You don't know what this one's really like yet. She's crazy, just like her father was."

My mother's words came as a shock to Marie. It wasn't the anger or the ranting that bothered her. It was the information about her father which was so upsetting. Marie had no memory of the rape. All she really knew of the man was what Mother had been telling her. For years she maintained the fiction that he was a good man who acted strangely because of some horrible disease. She had been raised to think kindly of him and had no idea that he died in the penitentiary. All she knew was what Mother told her and that wasn't what she was expressing now.

Marie was no longer thinking about her mother's rage. Her mind was filled with questions. It was the wrong time—the wrong circumstances.

Mother leaped from the table and charged toward Marie who realized she should try and flee. She raced to her bedroom, slamming the door in Mother's face. Mother pounded on the door, cursing and yelling, while Marie leaned against it, using her weight to hold it shut.

For several minutes Mother pounded while Marie held herself rigid against the door. Then Marie decided to stop protecting herself. She was overwhelmed with remorse for what had happened to Miriam and shocked by the comments about Father. She stepped away from the door and went over to the bed, rolling herself into a ball in an effort to protect herself from whatever violence was coming as Mother burst through the entrance.

Mother raced across the room, leaped onto the bed, and began pounding Marie with her fists. She saw Marie's head was exposed and reached up and bit Marie on the face as hard as she could. It felt like she was trying to bite through to the skull.

My stepfather ran into the room, grabbing my mother and pulling her from Marie.

Marie lay on the bed after everyone left, the door to her room closed. She didn't cry or move. She told herself it didn't matter; it didn't hurt. No one had ever loved her before so why should the hatred she had seen change anything. They weren't her family anymore. Not the way she imagined a family should be.

For the next several days the family was tense with one another. No one spoke much to Marie who returned to doing her chores as always. At first, Miriam didn't speak to her at all, then grunted in acknowledgment of her sister's presence. But gradually, as time passed, they began to speak.

One day Miriam went to her dresser drawer and brought out a small white box. She handed it to Marie, saying, "It was going to be a surprise for your birthday. Your birthday's not till tomorrow, but with all that's happened . . . Well, here. This is for you."

Marie took the box, opened it, and discovered a pretty red wallet. As she took it out of the box, Miriam said, "Open it. The surprise is inside!"

Inside were the photographs of herself with Walter.

The day that changed my life was no different from any other for Linda. It was 1954. I was twelve. Linda had had enough of the mink ranch.

She had been skipping school on and off for weeks. What Linda didn't know as she wandered the farmland was that this time, when the school called Mother to report Linda truant, Mother had had all she could take. This time she called the juvenile division of the police department. She told them that Linda was incorrigible. She could no longer get Linda to behave and she wanted the juvenile authorities to take charge of her child.

Linda frequently went to a girl friend's house when she played hookey, and the day Mother called the detectives was no exception. The officers tried that address first and were fortunate in surprising Linda. Even when she realized she was being placed under arrest and would be taken to a juvenile detention center, she made no effort to resist. The institution couldn't be any worse than her own home. Besides, if she didn't like the place, she could always go back in my mind and let one of the others take control.

The county's Juvenile Hall, where Linda was taken, was a small building meant for temporarily holding children no matter what their crimes had been.

Many times children were brought there for status offenses—"crimes" which were not considered against the law once you were of full legal age. Linda's truancy from school was a status offense, for example. So was staying out on the streets past the hour the city leaders had decided should be curfew for children. At the same time, Juvenile Hall was temporary home for children who were criminals by anyone's definition. These included burglars, dope peddlers, and even an occasional murderer.

There were ten cells for the juveniles and these were real cells, not rooms as you might expect for children who, in many cases, had done nothing more than run away from home. The cells were dirty, gray, solid cement and steel. The walls were plastered, though there was little of the white material visible to the eye. All of the plaster had been covered by the scrawls of countless children/inmates who had used graffiti as a means of asserting their unique identity in an uncaring world.

Fortunately the cells were meant to hold the children/inmates only while they slept, ate, or wanted some privacy. The rest of the time the children were allowed to have the run of the tightly locked facility. There was even a very small, totally enclosed yard where play was encouraged for an hour a day. Usually this meant tossing a basketball around, as there wasn't room for much else. We enjoyed it anyway, as it was the closest thing to freedom we knew there. All doors were locked, including the doors to our individual cells once we bedded down each night.

Each of the "inmates" wore blue jeans and a checkered, short-sleeved blouse supplied by the county. We also had access to games, puzzles, and similar amusements. But Linda preferred gossiping with the other teenagers.

Linda's hatred of the ranch and my mother was deeper than anyone realized, including herself. Juvenile Hall was a confining, tension-filled environment where personal freedom was nonexistent. Everything was controlled from the moment you awakened until you went to bed at night. There were strict rules to obey and no chance of going elsewhere. Yet this harsh environment, so typical of the institutions in which Linda would eventually spend much time, was a delight for her compared to life on the ranch.

Linda obeyed all the rules and showed no signs of rebelling, as some of the girls did. As a reward, she was made a kitchen worker by the elderly couple who lived in and cared for the detention center. This gave her access to what seemed like the most homelike section of the building. Because meals were needed for only a dozen or so people at a time, the kitchen was a large version of the one she had known at the ranch rather than an institutional facility.

The detention center held both boys and girls, though their sleeping quarters were separated. After Linda had been working in the kitchen just a few days, she overheard some Mexican boys planning an escape. They were going to steal a knife from the kitchen and use it as a weapon to force their way out. Since they didn't work in the kitchen as she did, their plans included forcing Linda to steal the knife for them. The boys were big and dangerous. Linda knew if she refused to steal the knife, she would be attacked by them and possibly badly hurt.

The detention center had a code of silence no different than the one my alter-personalities would encounter when, as adults, they went to prison. A prisoner did not tell the plans or deeds of another prisoner. You could witness a cold-blooded murder, but when the guards questioned you, you claimed no knowledge of it. Speaking up about such matters was an invitation to violence and, occasionally, death.

For Linda, the discipline she received was the closest thing to love she had known from the adults in her life. Someone actually cared where she was and what she did every minute of the day. They looked upon her as a real person, with thoughts and feelings worth understanding. It didn't matter that she was watched because the staff assumed she, like the others, might be dangerous. It didn't matter that the only reason people cared about her thoughts was because they were interested in monitoring them. To Linda, deprived of all affection ever since she was created during the brutal rape, prison meant love.

The detention center further established Linda's topsy-turvy moral code. Obviously her rebelling was something good to do because it resulted in the benefits she received from her confinement. Jail meant love, so why should she obey the dictates of society when being good meant your family ignored you and the other teens ridiculed you? It was better to be bad and get placed in a setting where everyone gave a damn about who you were and what you were doing.

She thrived at the detention center, keeping control of the body and showing no signs of rebellion.

Inevitably, Linda became tired of being isolated from the rest of the world. She would much rather be in the Juvenile Hall than on the ranch. But still, the place was a jail and none of the privileges she received could alter that fact. She knew that if she was ever given a chance, she too would flee the place.

One evening, while making a salad for dinner, a girl who worked in the kitchen with Linda noticed that the back door leading to the outdoor garbage area had been accidentally left unlocked. "It's open," the girl whispered to Linda. "Do you want to run for it?"

Linda gave no thought to the consequences of escaping. She was a prisoner and the open door led to freedom. She joined the other girl and together they raced outside and up the steep hill behind the Juvenile Hall.

Linda's friend decided they should go to her boyfriend for help. She was mistaken. As soon as they reached his apartment they were captured. It was only the first of many times I would be in and out of institutions.

After my return to the juvenile detention center, I was placed in another institution. Linda spent most of the time in control of my body while at Perkins, a prison for kids. She longed for respect from the people with whom she lived and, in the prison setting, she found it. She had given up trying to get my mother and stepfather's praise or affection. She had known for years that Miriam and Al would never think of her as anything more than the "baby" of the family. And she was ridiculed and humiliated by the rejection of the kids at school. Even Walter had turned away from Marie when she got into trouble with the law. He could date an "outsider" but not one who was amassing a criminal record. I was becoming more and more isolated and lonely.

Ultimately, it was determined that Linda was not repentant for the past and might continue her acts of truancy. The decision was made to send her to Los Guilocas, the State School for Wayward Girls. It was quite an "honor" for Linda. Normally admission to this "exclusive" facility is open only to young ladies who rob, steal, commit murder, or otherwise do violent physical harm to others. Thus a relatively innocent, troubled young teenager was being forced to adjust to living with the least desirable and most dangerous girls in the state.

Linda quickly became bored with the life at Los Guilocas. It was so large a facility that she no longer felt unique or special. She had no job or prestige coveted by the others. The inmate hierarchy was based on the seriousness of the crimes committed by the inmates before they were caught. Linda's actions had been so minor that her status was reduced. She eventually was so frustrated she returned to my mind and let Marie dominate.

The coldness of the surroundings was the first surprise. Marie found herself sitting on a chair in a small cell in the isolation ward of Los Guilocas.

I'm being punished, thought Marie. I'm being punished for the terrible things I must be doing during my blackouts. She had little memory of the previous jail experience and no memory of the judicial hearing which resulted in her being sentenced to prison. She had no way in which to evaluate the circumstance she found herself in. It was like dying and waking up in hell.

I'm no good, thought Marie. I'm dirty and sinful and evil. If I wasn't, why would I be here? I forget what happens to me because it's so bad that I'm ashamed. It's the only answer.

Gradually Marie came to accept her fate. She was certain something was wrong with her mind and equally certain she would never have the nerve to talk with someone about getting help. The rules of the state prevented girls from remaining in the prison once they reached legal adult status. But if Marie confessed her inner secrets, she was sure she'd be locked up for good. It was a possibility Marie could not risk having happen so she didn't reach out for the help she needed more and more desperately.

Marie managed to stay in charge of the body through most of the time at Los Guilocas. Linda recognized that if she was to get out as soon as possible, she had to keep out of trouble. Since she was lacking in status and knew her frustration would turn to disruptive action, she wisely let Marie retain control.

At the end of the year Marie was paroled. Mother drove out to pick her up. Marie was an ex-convict who had not yet reached her fourteenth birthday.

By the time Marie returned to the ranch, the character of my alter-personalities was well formed. Marie had become a frightend individual wishing desperately to pass as "normal." She was afraid of herself and the actions she took in the periods during which she had amnesia. She was mistrustful of friendship after being hurt by Walter's rejection, yet longed desperately for someone to care about her.

Linda, on the other hand, felt a new independence of spirit. She wanted respect and approval but she wasn't going to be hurt by my mother's denial of affection. She was determined to make her own way and to dominate every relationship. She was hard and bitter, convinced her sexual activities in the past would forever prevent normal relationships and determined to survive without them. She would take her pleasure when and where she could.

It was hard to make the adjustment from an inmate to an adolescent and I found myself increasingly on an emotional seesaw. The blackouts were more frequent and, worse, there was no one I could talk to. I was losing control, feeling myself more and more a victim of some horrible disease or mental illness that I could in no way understand, much less explain to someone else.

As the years of my early adolescence slipped by, I was less sure of who I was, where I was. Linda was becoming stronger, Marie more uncertain, and Charlene was there when I needed her, and I, Christina, of course, was buried deep in the graveyard of my mind.

An incident occurred when I was sixteen that served to push me further out of control.

The school year ended and Linda delighted in the new freedom of summer vacation. She had begun doing physical labor on the farm, an activity she enjoyed. Being physical helped her relieve her aggressions.

Linda was riding a tractor, digging deep trenches in which to bury dead mink in compliance with health department regulations when Mother told her the "good" news. There was going to be a family reunion of sorts in a few days. Al, who had enlisted, was returning from navy training. He would be bringing some friends and they would sleep on sleeping bags in a room just off the tool shed. Al, however, was going to be permitted to share my bedroom.

Linda was tired from working the tractor the first night the boys were at the ranch. They were out drinking and seeking excitement where they could find it. All Linda wanted to do was watch a little television, then go to bed at eight thirty. She knew Al might disturb her when he came in later, but that was a chance she'd take. At least she'd get some sleep by going to bed so early.

Al had been away from home long enough that Linda was accustomed to going to bed with almost no clothing on. She wore only underpants, letting the sheet or the blankets keep her warm. She was dressed this way from force of habit that first night that Al was out drinking.

It was late when Al returned home. His face was flushed and his breath was sour. He lurched into Linda's bedroom, fumbled with his clothing, and removed his pants. Then he walked over to Linda's bed, pulled down the blanket, and tried to work his body on top of hers.

The ranch was in an isolated area, off the main highways and in a community too small to attract a criminal element. Linda always felt safe from harm at home and was unconcerned when she was awakened by the touch of someone's body. She assumed whoever was there meant no harm and had stumbled against her in the dark.

"Wrong bed, buddy. This one's occupied," said Linda groggily. She didn't bother opening her eyes.

"Hold still," said Al.

"What are you doing?" exclaimed Linda, suddenly alert. Al was straddling her body, pulling off her underpants. "Stop it! Leave me alone!"

"It won't take very long. I'll be done before you know it." Al's words were slurred. His eyes were half-closed slits he seemed unable to focus. He had positioned himself in such a way that his knees pressed against the blanket covering Linda's legs and prevented Linda from kicking. His hands held her arms and he leaned forward so his body weight kept her pinned. His angle was such that she couldn't get free. When he was done, he left the room, sleeping off his drunk in a different part of the house rather than risking retaliation.

That was all that Linda could stand. It was time for her to divorce herself from the family. But it would be another year before Linda could make good her "escape." And then it would prove to be Marie rather than Linda who took the first step.

5
WEDDING-BELL BLUES

Mother had become aggressively flirtatious with all the men around her by the time I was approaching my seventeenth birthday. Whether or not she had affairs, I never knew. If she did, she was discreet.

Mother was jealous of Marie and Miriam when they were going through their teenaged years. She resented Marie's attractive figure and the blond hair that drew compliments. Whenever Mother went someplace where men were present, she'd try and flirt with them, dominating the conversation. She wore tight clothing and added more makeup.

Each morning one of Mother's tasks was to drive to the Santa Cruz fish wharf where she would obtain fresh fish heads from the day's cleaned catch. These were used in the making of mink feed and her trips were a high point of the day for her. She would joke with the fishermen and dock workers, flaunting her body and delighting in their obscene suggestions.

One of the dock workers was a Portuguese-American named Guido Quarro. He was a handsome youth, five years older than me, six feet three inches tall with naturally curly golden blond hair. His blue eyes were unusually large in contrast to his narrow face and Romanesque nose. His body was well developed and he took pride in his physical strength.

Guido was spoiled by his mother. Her only other child, Guido's brother, had been killed in an accident when Guido was six. His mother concentrated her attention on the surviving son, giving him anything he wanted. By the time he had grown to manhood, her indulgences were extremely lavish, for she had amassed great wealth.

Guido was somewhat of a "mamma's boy" and was in-secure about his manhood. He dedicated himself to proving that he was stronger and more physical than other men, taking on challenges which would test what he felt were the proper attributes for manliness.

His mother worked as a maid when she first came to the United States, saving all the money she could. After her mar-riage, she and her husband began investing in real estate, care-fully studying each community in which property was located to determine how quickly it might be resalable at a profit. They were extremely successful with their efforts and soon added a restaurant to their holdings. For the next twenty years, Guido's mother ran the restaurant and the couple con-tinued investing in real estate. They became extremely wealthy, though Guido's mother never let this influence her life. She regularly worked sixteen to twenty hours a day in the restau-rant, cooking, planning menus, and overseeing all the tasks which had to be done.

My mother was impressed with Guido the moment she met him. He was working as a commercial fisherman because he felt the life was rugged and "manly," whereas the family real estate or restaurant ventures were things a woman could handle. She invited him to the ranch to talk with Jacob. Once he arrived, however, he became immediately enchanted with Marie.

I'm nothing, thought Marie. I'm reasonably attractive but nobody cares about that. Mother says I'm worthless and she's probably right. Half the time I can't remember where I've been or what I've done the day before.

So why is this guy interested in me? He's rich. He's been all over the world with the marines. Why does he want to date me?

Marie was shocked by Guido's asking her to the drive-in

movies, even though they doubled at the drive-in with Mother and Jacob. He timidly held her hand, which proved another surprise. For all his efforts at proving his manliness, he seemed almost as shy as she was when it came to interpersonal relationships. Other guys she dated tried to paw her body, but not Guido. He was extremely handsome in his custom-tailored clothes and there was nothing sissified about him. Yet he acted as though Marie was something to be touched gently and with respect, like a crystal statue that might break if too much pressure was applied when holding it.

After several weeks of courtship, Guido took Marie to meet his mother. Natalie Quarro was a small, olive-complexioned woman whose frail appearance and smooth face belied the tireless work she had done all her adult life. Barely five feet tall, she seemed more like a child than the mother of a man as tall and powerful as Guido.

Marie quickly realized the importance of her visit to meet Natalie. Guido was following an Old World custom; he had never before brought a girl home to meet his mother. His bringing Marie was a way of letting his mother know this was a prospective marriage partner. She immediately approved, welcoming Marie as a daughter.

The idea of marrying so young had never occurred to Marie. She was still in high school and enough of a loner that Guido was her first serious romance. However, after all the put-downs concerning her time in jail and the way she was ostracized from clubs at school, it pleased her to see the envy in the other students' eyes when Guido picked her up in his expensive new car.

This guy's not to be believed, thought Linda. She was aware of the romance between Guido and Marie and she liked the idea of going off with him. He was handsome and rich and, most of all, could get her away from the ranch. But he was also "square."

Take the night Linda decided to see what he might be

like for sex. She took control of the body when Guido and Marie were parked near the ranch. Though Marie was reserved, despite the fact that they were engaged, Linda was determined to arouse him until he wanted her. As they kissed passionately, Linda started rubbing his chest with her hand, then worked it inside his shirt and against his bare skin. She unbuttoned the shirt, then dropped her hand to his pants. She could feel his arousal and was reaching to undo his zipper when he abruptly pushed her back.

"No!" said Guido, his face flushed and his stiffened penis pressing hard against his pants.

First time I saw a guy who didn't want to get his rocks off when he had the chance, thought Linda. But it hardly mattered. Linda had a ticket to escape. Marie could do the wifely duties. For once, the two personalities wanted the same thing.

Wedding plans were made. As the date drew closer, Marie decided she should tell Guido about her past, though not about her blackouts. She had avoided mentioning her time in the juvenile prison, and no one in her family brought up the subject. However, she was determined that if she was going to marry, the marriage should be based on trust and mutual understanding. She would tell Guido everything, a plan she explained to her parents before mentioning anything to her fiancé. Both Mother and Jacob were furious.

"You're lucky anyone wants you, the way you act," said Mother. "And especially a guy that rich and good-looking. He'll never speak to you again if you tell him about your past. Keep your big mouth shut and thank your lucky stars you found him."

Mother seemed to have a special interest in keeping Marie engaged to Guido. She asked as though she, too, desired him and was living vicariously through her daughter. She bleached her hair blond so it would be the same color as

Marie's and she began wearing skin-tight clothing, again emulating her daughter's form of dress. However, while Marie had the shape to look attractive in such outfits, Mother was enough overweight that she looked like a sausage about to split through its casing.

Marie reluctantly agreed with her parents. She didn't mention her past to him, nor did anyone else. Throughout the marriage he would think of her background as being "pure."

The marriage took place in September of 1959, Mother signing for Marie who was not yet of legal age. After the honeymoon, the couple returned to live near Natalie, and Marie went to work in the family restaurant, learning to cook.

As the days passed, Marie began to know Guido and realized that with all his looks and his money, he was not the man she expected. He was cold, withdrawn, and a loner. He loved Marie as much as he could love anyone, but he preferred to be wandering the hills, hunting and fishing by himself rather than spending time with his wife. His co-workers, keenly aware of his personality, called him "the ice man" and Marie understood why. However, despite her growing disillusionment, Marie became pregnant soon after the marriage and delighted in the attention she received as an expectant mother.

It was the end of May, 1960, when Marie went into labor. She had been seeing a doctor Mother recommended, a semi-competent individual who made no effort to prepare Marie for what birth would be like. He kept talking about how she would "naturally" do the right thing, the baby would come quickly, and she would know greater happiness than she had ever known before. Yet when he said the supposedly reassuring words, he sounded as though he was reading them from a prepared speech. He was abrupt and spent no time explaining the physical and emotional trauma, common to all births, which she would experience. Perhaps this wouldn't have been so bad with an older, more knowledgeable woman, but Marie was still a child herself and the thought of birth and impending motherhood frightened her.

The first pains of labor felt to Marie as though a knife was carving widening circles in her flesh. Thousands of tiny spears jabbed her stomach and she wanted to scream in agony. Each time the pain would reach a point where Marie thought she could endure no more, and then it stopped. She fought for breath, sobbing from the shock and fear, then tensely waited for the next wave which came after shorter and shorter intervals. Since Charlene had always been there to endure, it was difficult for Marie to deal with the pain.

Marie heard someone screaming, the voice growing louder and louder until the sound seemed to engulf her like a blanket, smothering all other voices in the room. Slowly she realized she was the one who was screaming. Then a second voice, softer and higher-pitched, joined the wailing cries which echoed from the room. This second sound was that of a new life—her baby son. As the pain began to ease and her eyes focused through the tears, she could see the nurse holding the tiny body in the air. She started to smile, then closed her eyes and drifted to sleep.

At first Marie was caught up in the excitement everyone in the family felt about the birth. Guido was moved at the idea of being a father and his emotionalism deeply touched Marie. She also liked the presents and the joy she shared with Mother, who had formerly been so distant. But after the first week at home, Marie's attitude changed.

It's as though she decided to skip a generation of our family, thought Marie. She never had time to give me attention when I was growing up. She never sang to me or touched me with affection. I was either something in the way to be kicked aside or kept out of sight and forgotten. She had love for her mother and she has love for my baby. But she turns away from me. How can she take the child into her heart and deny its mother?

To add to the pressure Marie was feeling, she and

Guido had taken the new baby to the ranch for the first three weeks after its birth. The familiar surroundings kept the memory of her own upbringing constantly in Marie's mind. The contrast in affection made her increasingly depressed with each passing day and she was greatly relieved when Guido said it was time they returned to their own home and establish a sense of normalcy.

Marie thought she could control her emotions when she was in her own home, but that was not the case. Her mother continued to visit the baby every day.

"Mother, if you keep coming down and playing with Guido when he should be sleeping, it keeps him awake later on. You can go home and not worry about him but I have to stay here while he's crying and cranky. You're turning his natural schedule upside down and it's making it impossible for me to have a normal day."

"You selfish little brat!" said Mother angrily. "After all the heartache you've caused me over the years, you have the nerve to tell me I shouldn't be visiting my first grandchild. Well, you're no longer a child. You're a mother, and that means your time will never be your own again. My interruptions are pretty minor and you just better get used to them. There'll be plenty more children and you're going to have to be more flexible whether you like it or not!"

Marie was outraged. Her mother was talking about children, not just the one baby. She had never paid any attention to Marie when she was growing up, but suddenly she was planning Marie's adult life.

"This is my son," said Marie, taking baby Guido from Mother's arms. "And this is my house which I want you to leave right now!"

Mother angrily walked from the house as Marie watched, holding her baby. Her body was shaking and she felt weak. She quickly took the infant to its bedroom, laid him in his crib, and closed the door.

Guido began to cry. Marie stood outside the door, her body tense. The crying grew louder, more intense. God, that noise is upsetting, Marie thought, putting her hands to her ears and walking over to the couch. In a minute, when she calmed down, she would go back into the nursery and comfort her baby. But right now, all she felt was frustration. She recognized her feelings of jealousy toward the baby who had won Mother's affection when Marie could not.

Suddenly Marie seemed to stare at the wall, her eyes glazed, her hands still covering her ears. Then her eyes grew bright and a half smile crossed her lips. Her hands came away from her ears and she rose to her feet.

Listen to that snot-nosed little bugger wail, thought Linda, looking toward the nursery. Why the hell anyone has brats like that is beyond me. Crying like that isn't going to get anywhere with me.

Linda walked over to the television set and turned it on. But there wasn't anything interesting and the crying made it hard to concentrate.

Linda moved to the bedroom, stood listening for a moment, then threw the door open and walked to the crib. Guido stared up at her, startled by her presence. His breathing was labored from all the crying but he no longer uttered a sound. His tiny eyes tried to focus on Linda and he was obviously tense. He seemed to sense the potential menace of the woman in front of him.

"She get you walking yet?" asked Linda, taking the baby from the crib and placing him on the floor. Her hands were rough, but Guido didn't cry. His body was rigid and, when he was on the ground, he tried to curl into a fetal position, as though to protect himself from attack.

"Go on. Let me see you do your stuff. Walk around the room. You're supposed to be so damned special, that's the least you can do."

Guido didn't move.

Linda took her foot and touched Guido's stomach. The baby stiffened and gasped but didn't cry.

"You look like a football," she said, bringing her foot back then kicking forward, catching the infant in the stomach and sending him rolling across the floor. His head bounced against the carpet and his body struck the far wall before he stopped.

"How do you like that?" asked Linda, her voice rising in pitch. "All my life I've been kicked around by that bitch grandmother of yours but you don't know anything about that, do you?" She moved menacingly toward the tiny, badly bruised body on the floor. "I'll show you what it's like to get kicked around. I'm going to kick you all over this floor until you hurt as bad as I did."

Linda brought her foot back, then started a rapid kick with far more force than the first one. There was a smile on her lips and her eyes seemed to sparkle with all the happy radiance of a girl attending her first big dance.

Just before Linda's shoe struck the baby, her foot stopped in mid-flight. Her face became a glazed mask and her body was rigid. Then she slowly eased her foot back down on the carpet and swiftly bent over the infant who relaxed and started to cry softly.

"Don't cry, little Guido," said Charlene, her voice soothing and gentle. She had been aware of Linda's actions and knew Marie could not regain control of the body soon enough to prevent the baby from being badly hurt or killed. She realized that if the baby was to have a chance at life, she would have to expand her role from that of someone meant to endure my body's physical and emotional pain to that of a rescuer. It was a role she would have to play many times.

Charlene's hands caressed the baby's forehead, then

quickly began feeling his entire body. She felt his bones and examined him for injuries. There was a chance Linda had broken a rib or one of his delicate arms or legs.

When Charlene satisfied herself that baby Guido was physically unharmed, she quickly receded back into my mind.

Marie looked about the room. She was in the nursery, though her last memory was of being on the couch. Somehow Guido had crawled or been carried from his bed to the spot on the floor where she had found him. Yet he couldn't get out of the bed by himself and she didn't remember lifting him from it.

It's happening again, Marie thought to herself. I'm forgetting things. And this time it's affecting my baby. If I don't get control, I don't know what might happen. He could crawl out of the house and get hurt and I'd never know it. Oh, my God . . . My God . . .

Marie started to cry as she hugged baby Guido close against her breasts. Her tears mingled with those of her infant, each of them expressing their fears of a life they didn't understand.

My second child, a daughter, was born in 1962. She was a quiet, well-behaved child and offered little trouble. Again the family fussed over the infant but not to the same degree as with Guido, Junior. Neither my mother nor Natalie looked upon daughters as being as special as sons. There was less reason for my alter-personalities to resent the baby or be jealous of it. As a result, Linda never attempted to hurt the child.

Guido seemed quite stable and mature during the first years of marriage. However, Guido had his own emotional difficulties. He never was certain how a man should behave, and his reactions when placed in circumstances that violated his sense of proper manhood were quite unpleasant. One incident in particular alerted Marie that her marriage was not going to last for many more years.

It was early one morning when my brother, Al, called Marie's house. His driver's license had expired and he had to renew it right away. Marie agreed to help him out.

Marie was concerned about who would take care of the two children. Even though Guido had the day off, he always considered such tasks to be her job, and she had always gone along with him. She called Mother, but Mother had to make a feed run and couldn't help out. Natalie was busy in the restaurant as well. The only person left was Guido.

"You know I don't know anything about taking care of the children," said Guido.

"Then it's time you learned," said Marie. "They're your children, too."

Guido reluctantly agreed to the arrangement. However, the situation proved more involved than Marie had anticipated.

It was close to two in the afternoon when Marie and Al returned to Marie's house. Marie was shocked to see Natalie's car parked in the drive. There was no way Natalie would have taken time off from the restaurant unless something serious had happened. Marie pulled quickly to the curb, leaped from the car, and ran into the house.

The two children were in different rooms, crying loudly. Marie went to the nursery first. The baby was standing in the crib, stark naked. Oatmeal covered the crib, the floor, and part of the wall. Even worse, there was a large brown object on the blanket. To Marie's horror she realized it was a bowel movement. The baby had been without a diaper and had made a mess where she lay.

Natalie entered the nursery, carrying little Guido. She looked confused and a little frightened.

Suddenly Marie sensed someone else had entered the room. She turned and saw her husband holding a washcloth he was bringing to his mother.

"You . . ." snarled Guido. "Just where the hell have you been? You were out having a good time while I was going crazy with those damn kids."

"What sort of man are you, Guido? You're carrying on like I abandoned you. My God, I was only gone a couple of hours."

Guido wasn't willing to listen to anything. He shoved Marie out the front door, spun her around, and kicked her in the rear, sending her sprawling into the flowerbed.

"I hate you, Guido," said the shocked Marie. "You're just like every other stinking person on this earth. You take and take and take but you never give. I thought you loved me, but you don't give a damn about me or your children."

Guido stared at his wife as she lay in the dirt; his breathing was accompanied by great sobbing sounds. He was part enraged, part frustrated, and part ashamed of himself as a man. He turned away and left the house, hurrying down the street.

Although Marie hadn't told Guido, she was pregnant when he kicked her. She feared she would lose the baby, but neither the kick nor the fall had been hard enough to damage her child.

The third baby, born in 1963, was also a girl. This time there were problems, however. The baby had colic, a periodic severe pain that she could neither understand nor control. She cried frequently and seldom got more than an hour or two's sleep at a time without being awakened by the discomfort. Guido remained irresponsible about his children.

Early one morning, Marie called the pediatrician after her baby had an unusually troubled night.

The doctor gave Marie an appointment for that afternoon. Guido refused to take off from work to help her.

"Mother? This is Marie." She felt tense, her stomach churning. She did not want to be calling Mother for help but there was no alternative. "I have to take the baby to the doctor. Her colic was worse last night and he's going to try some new medicine. I've been up for hours and I don't think I can handle the baby, the driving, and the other two kids. Do you think you could give me a hand?"

Even over the telephone, Marie felt the woman's presence dominating her home. "I raised just as many children as you've got and I never once had the problems you keep talking about. Sometimes I think you just don't know what you're doing. You're more of a baby than the children. If you weren't so empty-headed and irresponsible, you wouldn't be having so much trouble. You bring these things on yourself, you know. You should just thank your lucky stars that a fine, handsome man like Guido somehow managed to find you attractive and . . ."

When Marie finally hung up the phone, she felt nauseated. She felt as though she had swallowed a vial of acid that was slowly eating the walls of her stomach. There was a painful aching sensation above one eye and her body was tense. In the other room she could hear the faint crying of the baby just beginning to react to her latest discomfort from the colic.

I've got to lie down for a moment, Marie told herself, heading for the couch. I'm tense and exhausted. I've got to lie down and get control of myself. I've got to . . .

Linda rose from the couch.

The baby's crying was growing louder. The sound was painful to Linda and she winced from the shrillness of the sobbing.

"Asshole has to take this shit but not me," said Linda, looking about the room.

Linda spotted the container in which Marie bathed the baby. "I'll drown the little shit," said Linda. "Everybody knows how easy it is for a baby to drown in bath water."

She filled the container with warm water, whistling to

herself as she worked. She carefully checked the temperature to be certain it was just right for the infant's tender skin. If she got it too hot it might burn the baby and that would be a giveaway that something was wrong. Marie was too careful a mother to let her baby get injured by overheated bath water. Linda had to be certain everything was as normal as possible so there would be no question about the "accident."

The baby was crying louder. Linda walked into the nursery and approached the crib.

Linda set the infant in the water. Its body was completely submerged but its head floated so the nose and mouth were above the surface. She put her hand on the baby's chest and forced it entirely under the water. The baby thrashed about for a few moments, as water slowly replaced the air in its lungs. Then it was still. Linda removed her hand and watched with satisfaction as the body remained below the surface. She would leave it there another couple of minutes to be certain it was dead, then call the fire department.

Charlene rushed over and quickly took the tiny, unmoving infant from the bath water. She turned the baby upside down and hit her on the back. Her approach was crude but effective.

Linda knew of the existence of Marie but not of Charlene. She never realized who it was that was fighting for control of the body during those occasions when she was pushed aside in Charlene's frantic haste to handle whatever danger confronted Marie or her babies.

The baby began crying, and Charlene took it in her arms, crooning softly. She felt no emotion toward the child. It was a job to her, a role for this life. When the baby was again safe, Charlene went back to the recesses of my mind and a rather confused Marie was again in charge.

That afternoon Mother came by the house to help Marie take the baby to the doctor. The pediatrician discovered that there were several tiny fractures on the baby's feet and legs. They were probably caused by Linda's rough handling while carrying the baby to the bath. So Marie had to face the fact that her baby had been hurt during one of her blackouts. What kind of mother was she?

Shortly after the attempted murder of my third child, Linda abandoned thoughts of killing the babies but decided she needed more excitement in life. She had taken control far less frequently than she liked and felt it was time to have some fun. She took charge of the body and immediately instituted changes in the family life-style which shocked Guido and caused the marriage to deteriorate.

"I'm a redhead," said Linda. "You should have hair the color of how you feel and I feel like a redhead." She had also purchased a totally new wardrobe several sizes too small as an incentive to keep on a diet. Within weeks she had lost twenty-five pounds and was slinking about the house in tight pants and blouses that were more revealing than anything Marie had ever considered wearing. She also let her nails grow long and kept them brightly painted and sharply pointed. Rings were placed on every finger and several bracelets adorned each wrist.

"I want to get a job," said Linda. Several months had passed since she began the transformation in life-style, and there was constant tension in the house.

"You mean you want to spend more time at the restaurant?"

"I mean a job. My own job. Not being a part-time slave for that bitch of a mother of yours. She has the biggest mouth in the smallest body I've ever seen."

Guido held his temper. Ordinarily such words would have led to a fight but Guido had become accustomed to Linda's way of talking and the fact that she refused to answer to the name "Marie." He was spending less and less time at home, preferring to be with his co-workers or in a bar somewhere rather than trying to deal with the person his wife had become. "What sort of 'real job'?" he asked. "The way you look, you're more like a streetwalker than the mother of my babies."

"There's a drive-in looking for a car hop. I saw the ad in the paper. You can make real good tips that way."

"What do you need tips for? I make plenty of money for both of us. Look at all those rings you're wearing. Whose money do you think paid for them? You make a couple bucks an hour at one of those places and you're doing pretty good. That's not going to pay for rings and bracelets."

"But it'll be my money and not something you gave me. Besides, I've already applied for the job and I go to work Friday. New girls have to work the weekends but at least the tips are better then."

Guido told Linda what he thought of her. He argued then begged, then pleaded. The marriage was rapidly coming to an end, yet he couldn't comprehend what had caused so many changes so suddenly.

A few days later, Linda went to see an attorney about getting a divorce. She insisted he call her Linda but used Marie's name when signing the papers since that was the name she had used when she got married. The divorce was not contested by Guido.

6
MEN AND MADNESS

Bowling alleys were the centers for leisure-time activity in the California community where Marie lived after her divorce. Following her divorce from Guido, Marie, almost twenty-three, took a job as a waitress in the cocktail lounge of one of the most popular bowling alleys in her community. The hours were long but the tips were excellent and she made enough money to pay for an apartment for herself and the three children. Guido also paid child support of $200 a month which enabled her to hire baby sitters while she was away from home.

Marie fully accepted the divorce even though she couldn't remember some of the events discussed in the legal papers that were filed. She knew her marriage had fallen apart and it was a relief to be free from the frequent arguments with Guido. She hoped that when she was on her own and more relaxed, her memory might improve as well. She was anxious to rid herself of the blackouts and periods of lost time. Perhaps living away from Guido would help.

Linda was seldom in control of my body during the early evening hours. That was when the bar was packed and orders came rapidly and endlessly. Let that bitch Marie run her tail off, thought Linda. I can wait until it's quiet and the men left are looking for some action.

During the time she worked at the bowling alley, Marie gravitated toward the lonely, quiet men who often came to the lounge around the dinner hour. They were loners— unmarried, widowed, or divorced.

One of the regulars was a man named Craig Randall. He was a shy, quiet man who felt he had been destined for death from the day he was born.

Marie became increasingly friendly with Craig. He wasn't handsome like some of the men, though he was appealing. He was a couple of inches short of six feet, trim and athletic-looking.

"What happened to your wrists?" Marie asked Craig late one afternoon.

Craig stared at the table for a moment, not answering. Then he took a sip of his drink and looked at Marie sadly. "I tried to kill myself once."

Slowly Craig explained. The incident had occurred when he was married, a few months after his wife had given birth to a son. He came home early from work and discovered his wife in bed with his brother. To make matters worse, the affair, which he had never suspected, had been going on long enough so that Craig was worried that he hadn't really fathered his child. He became so depressed he didn't want to continue living.

Marie was deeply touched by Craig's story. She had the same hopeless feelings herself, though she couldn't imagine killing herself. When he asked her to date him that night, she accepted.

It was a decision she would have cause to regret.

Craig was a very dependent individual and, within a few weeks' time, was begging Marie to marry him. She didn't want to get married; she was trying to make a life for herself, and the pressure threw her into a tailspin.

I don't want to get married, thought Marie. I've done that and it just doesn't work for me. I had a guy with everything a woman could want—money, fancy clothes, a beautiful house—but I was miserable. I'd rather go it alone with the kids, even if it is hard to make ends meet.

Why can't Craig be happy the way we are? We see each other almost every day as it is. Why does he have to keep proposing marriage? I want my freedom. I'm not ready for a permanent commitment, even if we do have so much in common.

The kids are the only problem right now. Every time I get a good sitter, she leaves me because of the way she says I'm behaving. The last one claimed I came in three hours later than I promised and was drunk and abusive. She said I called her a two-bit whore, but I've never used such language in my life.

Tears came to Marie's eyes. I don't know who I am half the time. If I'm going crazy, why is it happening so slowly? Crazy people laugh and shriek and tear off their clothing in the middle of Main Street. I haven't done that yet. At least no one says I have. So why do they say I do things I know I couldn't be doing? And why can't I remember better? How can I be a decent mother if I don't remember what I said or did just hours before?

The telephone rang. When Marie answered it, she discovered it was a girl who had gone to school with Craig and married one of his friends. Marie knew her only casually, yet the girl felt she could call Marie for advice about an unusually personal problem.

"It's Mort," wailed the girl. "He's been seeing someone else. All the time he's holding me in bed, telling me how much he loves me, the rotten son of a bitch has been seeing someone else. I don't know what to do. I don't know where to turn. Marie, you've got to help me. You've got to . . ."

Linda looked at the telephone Marie had been holding. Craig's friend was asking her what to do about her husband.

"Why don't you get yourself a sex manual?" said Linda, her voice cruelly harsh. "Obviously balling you doesn't keep him happy so maybe you need a few lessons. Men don't stray if they get enough action at home."

The girl on the other end of the telephone was shocked. She had turned to Marie for help, not insults. She started to curse as Linda hung up the receiver.

I've got to get rid of Marie, thought Linda. I'm sick of the way she acts like a doormat for every creep with a hard-luck story. She takes darn-fool jobs and works her butt off for peanuts. And those damned brats of hers. I'm sick of their runny noses, their puking, and all the other crap. If I had succeeded in killing them, we'd all be a lot better off.

Linda had tried alcohol for the first time at twenty-one. She liked the way liquor helped her forget her problems. She also had a tremendous capacity for holding alcohol. The constant surge of adrenaline through her body counteracted the numbing effects of liquor and she could continue drinking long after her companions had passed out at the table. Heavy drinking quickly became a way of life.

Marie tried liquor several months after Linda first started drinking. She had been experiencing the sick headaches and nausea of hangovers for some time without realizing why.

Marie had less capacity for liquor than Linda, but she, too, quickly began to drink too much. As Linda became an alcoholic, her body changed subtly. She felt the need for a drink with increasing frequency. Marie was in charge, this craving continued, making it easy for her to slip into a pattern of excessive drinking almost at once. It might be said that because of Linda, Marie became an alcoholic with her very first sip.

I've got to destroy Marie, thought Linda, rising from the table where she was sitting. She went to the bathroom and began filling the bathtub with hot water. Then she took a razor blade from the medicine cabinet and made an incision in each wrist. She used a quick cutting motion, pushing the blade as deep as she thought necessary. Then she plunged her bleeding wrists into the hot water and receded into my mind.

Charlene withdrew her wrists and grabbed some towels. Desperately she tried applying pressure to the wounds to stop the bleeding. She managed to slow the flow, but the towels continued filling with blood. The loss of fluid was affecting her body as well. She was light-headed and knew she would soon lose consciousness. The blood coming from her wrists was slowing but she could not completely stop the flow. As she looked desperately about for additional towels, she lost consciousness.

Marie awakened on her back on a steel hospital bed, staring up at graying white walls.

A male attendant entered the room and smiled at Marie. He carried a glass of water with a straw in it. "I see you've awakened," he said. "I thought you might like a drink."

"What I'd like is to get untied. Why are my wrists like this? And how did I get here?"

He looked at her oddly. "You should remember that," said the orderly, bending the straw so Marie could sip the water. "You're the one who slashed your wrists."

Slashed my wrists? thought Marie. This is insane. I've got to talk with somebody. I've got to tell somebody what's happening to me. I'm in a hospital. Surely there's a psychiatrist who can help me.

The children ... If I tell a psychiatrist about all that's been happening over the years, they'll take the children and put them in a foster home. Then they'll lock me away forever. They'll keep me in an institution until they think I'm well enough to leave. And if they decide I'll never be safe on the outside ...

No, I've got to go on like before. I've got to lie about what happened and say whatever words will get me released in the shortest possible time. Maybe if I tell them I've been unusually depressed. That's it. I'll just say that I've been going through a particularly bad time and I lost my head. I never tried suicide before and I'll never try it again.

That's what I'll do. I'll lie so I can keep the kids with me. And from now on, I'm going to stay aware of what's happening to me. In the future, I'm not going to forget and find myself with slashed wrists. I'm going to make it on my own.

Craig had come to the hospital as soon as Mother called to tell him what happened. He had been waiting during all the hours Marie was unconscious, and he entered the room only after one of the nurses asked Marie if she wanted to see him. The restraints had been removed and Marie was sitting on the side of her bed, her robe and blankets wrapped around her. She was pale and dizzy from loss of blood but happy to see him.

Gradually the full story came out. Marie learned about the slashed wrists and the fact that she was on a seventy-two-hour hold. When someone attempted suicide, the doctor who treated the injuries could order the person held for three days in the psychiatric ward while tests were conducted to determine mental stability. This was the case with Marie.

It's finally happened to me, thought Marie. All these years I've feared being locked away and now they've gone and done it to me. They say they're going to give me a bunch of tests and I can go home if I pass. But what if I don't pass? What if I have one of my blackouts and do God-knows-what on the papers? How long can they keep me here? How long . . .

I've got to give Guido the children, thought Marie. I thought I could raise them. I thought I could give them the love and attention I never had as a child. I thought I could make up to them for the way their father acted before I left him. But how can I take care of them if I slash my wrists and never know it? One day I might hurt them or ignore them when they need me. Maybe I've already done it and don't remember. I can't risk that.

"So you can see we've got to get married right away. You need me to take care of you. You need me ..."

Marie turned her head toward Craig, aware of what he was saying for the first time. She heard his latest proposal of marriage and saw the concern in his eyes. She put her head against his shoulder and began crying softly.

Marie never relaxed during her three-day stay in the psychiatric ward, even though she knew she could not be kept longer than the minimum time. Craig had been talking constantly with the doctors and he convinced them that he would be able to take care of Marie. In addition, none of the tests she had taken seemed to indicate that anything was mentally wrong with Marie. Multiple personality is not detectable through standard psychological tests; each personality would score like a normal person, though the answers and psychiatric appraisal would be different for each one. Only by comparing the same test taken by each different personality could any mental problem be noticed by someone unaware he was dealing with a multiple personality.

Marie tried to remain calm the day she was released from the psychiatric ward. She walked at a controlled pace through the door that had always been locked to her during her stay. She tensed as she heard the key inserted in the lock and the bolt jammed home again behind her. Then she realized that she was no longer on the inside, no longer confined by that horrid sound. The lock was keeping her out, not holding her in. She exhaled, her body relaxing, and walked to the steps leading to the main section of the hospital and total freedom. Her pace quickened with each step until she was almost running.

I'm free! Marie thought to herself. She had been so sure they'd never let her out.

Marie burst through the front door of the hospital, knocking two interns off balance. They had to clutch each other to keep from falling, and Marie realized she had better slow down. She knew she must look like a crazy woman running, with her hair flying in the breeze and a huge grin on her face. They might return her to the ward on general principles. She slowed her step and continued at a more dignified rate.

There was a park nearby and Marie walked through, watching the squirrels scampering up and down trees, retrieving nuts people had thrown, then darting to and fro in the grass. She saw couples sitting under the trees. They were obviously in love and totally absorbed in each other. Cars moved along the streets. Cyclists rode down the bike paths. Birds flew overhead. Dogs romped in the high grass. And everywhere—fabulously, wonderfully, joyously, everywhere—all creatures were free.

I can't go back to that cage they call a psychiatric ward again. I can't discuss my problems and risk having them take away all this freedom. I don't want to ever again hear a key in a lock and know that my life is going to be limited to just four walls.

When Marie returned to Craig, he had a box containing two wedding rings which he held open in front of her. "You've got to marry me, Marie," he pleaded. "You love me; I know you do. And I'd do anything for you."

Though Craig kept begging her to marry him, Marie was adamant. She reasoned that she needed to have a life free of entanglements in order to keep the awful secret of her lost time to herself. Somehow the idea of marriage was bound up in her mind with absolute honesty. She had vowed to herself that she would never again marry a man she couldn't be completely honest with. It was a vow she was destined to break. But for the moment, she stuck to it.

She was, however, in dire need of close companionship.

It was for that reason she agreed to live with Craig.

A few months after Marie and Craig began living together, Marie discovered she was pregnant. The shock overwhelmed her.

Stupid, fucking bitch! Now she's gone and done it. First she has to trade one creep for another, and then she gets herself knocked up again.

Linda paced the floor, then grabbed her purse and headed for the door. Got to think. Got to go somewhere away from his home; his smell. Got to plan . . .

Linda drove to a liquor store and bought enough bottles to last for days. She was drinking more and more when she went out, and she had concluded that if ever she needed a drink, it was now.

Linda drove to a hotel and took a room. She spread the liquor bottles on the dresser, locked the door, then sat down and started drinking.

For the next three days, Linda drank until she lost consciousness.

While Linda was in a drunken stupor, Craig was desperately searching for Marie.

Finally, after three days, Craig located the hotel where Linda had registered. He paid her bill and was given a key to her room. He found her unconscious. Instead of feeling angry or disgusted, his heart went out to her. He wrapped her in a blanket, took her to the car, and brought her home to clean and care for her.

The baby was a girl who was born healthy and strong despite Linda's drinking spree at the start of the pregnancy. Craig and Marie named the child Tina; Craig began exerting even more pressure on Marie to marry him. "A baby should have a name," he said. "She needs a father who *is* a father in the eyes of the law. You've just got to marry me, Marie."

Six months after Tina's birth, Marie and Craig were married in a small Presbyterian church near where they were living. No one was particularly happy about the marriage —least of all Linda.

That does it! I'm through standing by and watching this shit. It's bad enough she lived with that whiny, limp-dicked creep. Now she's gone and married him and kept the kid. Well, hell, I've had enough.

Linda remembered a man named Jack Headley who had been a regular at the bowling alley lounge.

Jack didn't seem surprised by Linda's sudden appearance at his door. Apparently he was ready for anything at any time. He smiled, let her inside, and the two of them headed directly for the bedroom. They both were interested in the same thing and no conversation was necessary.

Linda never felt she was doing anything wrong in her frequent liaisons with Jack and others. Her sexual activity quickly became common knowledge among many of the men in the community where she was living. As a result, word eventually reached Craig, who was deeply hurt. While he had been saddened to the point of suicide the first time, he was now angry. He refused to be made a fool. He took a rifle, loaded it, and sat near the front door, waiting for his wife to come home.

". . . Whore! Slut!"

"Craig, we can't talk like this. All you're going to do is upset Tina and bring the neighbors running. Put down that rifle and let's sit together to discuss the problem. Nothing's so bad we can't talk it out."

Craig finally put away the rifle and went with Marie into the living room. As they talked, Marie gradually came to understand what was troubling her husband. The idea of her cheating on him shocked her. She wasn't that kind of person.

Yet what Craig said made sense out of other things that had been happening to her lately. When she was in the stores or on the street, a man would occasionally come over to her and make suggestive remarks about going to bed. Other men placed their hands on her rear or her breasts and were shocked when she slapped them. She knew she never did anything suggestive to lead them on, yet they all acted as though she had encouraged them in the past.

Insanity, thought Marie. My mind is gone. I'm living the lives of two different women, never remembering what I do when I go out somewhere.

After what seemed like hours of talking, Craig picked up his rifle, unloaded it, and put it away. Then he and Marie went to bed. She was deeply troubled and confused but she confided none of her fears to Craig. He wouldn't understand. How could he? She didn't understand herself.

Linda sat up in bed just moments after Marie had fallen asleep. She looked at Craig by her side and watched to see if his breathing was slow enough to indicate he was asleep. When she satisfied herself that he was, she carefully slid from the bed and put on a robe.

Nobody calls me a two-bit whore and gets away with it, especially not that creep Craig, thought Linda. She went to the window, opened it carefully so as to not make noise, then stepped through. There was a small shed in back where Craig kept tools and lumber. Linda walked to it, selected a heavy board, and carried it back through the window with her.

Craig stirred slightly but didn't awaken. Linda walked slowly over to the bed, raised the board high above her head, and shouted, "Call me a whore, will you?"

Craig stirred, shocked awake by Linda's raucous voice. He started to rise just as the board smashed down against his head. The edge caught his ear, slicing it partway off. He lost consciousness, bleeding profusely. Smiling happily, Linda returned to her "room" in my mind.

Marie was horrified by the bloody sight that greeted her eyes. As she drove Craig to the hospital for stitches, Marie realized she was capable of great violence she couldn't remember, actions counter to her normal moral code. She had to get help. She knew that. But from whom she did not know. Somehow she had to function as normally as she could until she could figure out where to turn.

Craig's job with the telephone company changed to a position which required he make fairly frequent trips out of town. Linda looked upon these occasions as times for celebration. She would go out with men, delighting in her freedom. Fortunately, Linda recognized that Marie's child, Tina, needed care. When she couldn't get a baby sitter, she bundled up Tina and took her with her. She had no love for the child but also no interest in hurting her—at least not yet.

One evening Linda located a baby sitter, then stopped by a bar where many of the telephone company employees went for entertainment. Within five minutes of ordering she was joined by a co-worker of Craig's, a man named Leonard Peters.

Linda had never met Leonard, though he knew Marie quite well. He was introduced to her when she and Craig were out for an evening. Len was the kind of man who radiated sex appeal and he had tried to pick up Marie in front of her husband. He knew the stories about Marie and was surprised when she reacted coldly.

"Hey, Marie, having a little fun while the old man's

out of town?" asked Len, sitting next to Linda.

Linda looked at Len and liked what she saw. He was almost six feet tall with broad shoulders, muscular arms, and a narrow waist. His jet-black hair, given an assist by dye after he started graying two years earlier, was kept shiny with an extra dab of Brylcreem. He was forty-two years old, nineteen years older than Linda, though he looked no older than thirty.

"The name is Linda and he's not my old man if you're talking about Craig." She smiled warmly. This was the first man she ever met whom she found totally arousing.

Linda suddenly realized Marie must have met this man at some time in the past. She would have to fake it, picking up his name and learning the way they first met from his conversation and the comments of others who came by to talk during the evening.

(Linda and Marie had a common problem with their memories. When one learned a particular fact, the other did not have it in her memory unless she came upon it separately. Marie was an avid student of geography, while Linda embarrassed herself at a party by trying to learn how many places a plane leaving the California coast would land before reaching Hawaii.)

Linda and Len left the bar and went to Linda's home. They went immediately to bed, Linda discovering a passion and sexual pleasure she never knew anyone could experience.

Len didn't stay the night but returned to Linda's house shortly after nine the next morning. He called first, claiming he was going to come by for doughnuts and coffee. But when he arrived, neither he nor Linda had any interest in food.

Craig returned and Linda receded in favor of Marie, who was genuinely pleased to see her husband. Linda was frightened that Len might want to meet with her at a time when Marie was in control of the body. She was determined to keep herself in charge of the body during the hours when Craig was at work. Len knew her husband's schedule and would only call when Craig was away.

Linda developed a passion that surprised her. If a day passed when she did not hear from Len, she became extremely depressed and began drinking heavily. As a means of being closer to him, Linda managed to become friendly with Len's wife. Then Len and his wife and Linda and Craig would make a foursome at shows, restaurants, and other places. Neither of the spouses suspected that they were being made party to an intense affair that would destroy both marriages. In fact, when Len's wife realized that another woman was becoming extremely important in her husband's life, it was to Linda that she confided her troubles. Naturally Linda was most understanding.

God, the last thing I need is some man dominating my life. I've always wanted to be on top of a relationship. Use 'em and lose 'em, that's the way I've always operated. Men are such stupid shits; all out for themselves.

But this is different. I've never met a man who could really turn me on like he does. He just has to come close and I want to wrap my legs around his body and ride his prick until I collapse from exhaustion. That man is not to be believed and I've got to have him full time.

But there's Craig. That sniveling, blubbering Jell-O mold of nothing is screwing up everything. Linda decided to introduce Marie to her lover. After having sex with Len, Linda would recede into my mind and let Marie take control.

Marie was frightened by Len at first. She had known him from the bar, which she and Craig occasionally visited, but she never wanted to be alone with the man. She was horrified to find herself with him and, even worse, in what was obviously a dating situation.

I function, thought Marie. I function very well. I get from day to day looking perfectly natural to everyone or I wouldn't still be walking the streets.

Maybe there's a logical explanation for all this and if I just asked the right person, he'd give it to me. Maybe I inwardly want to have an affair with Len and my amnesia is just a way of avoiding responsibility. I know I should be a faithful wife, yet I want Len too much to stay away from him. I . . .

How can I think this? It doesn't make sense at all.

Even if I'm right about my amnesia, how do I know for certain? Who do I ask? Where do I go? If I walk into the psychiatric ward, they'll refuse to treat me until I agree to voluntary commitment. Then, when I'm securely locked inside the walls, they'll declare me incompetent to judge my own affairs. Instead of being able to check myself out any time I want to leave, I'll have to stay until they say I can go. And that could be five years, ten years, God knows how many years.

Marie studied Len, who was reading a newspaper, periodically looking up to discuss some item of interest. She had not been close to a man other than Craig since her marriage. She forced herself to stop worrying about how she had come to be in the coffee shop and started looking at Len objectively. She was impressed with him.

Linda decided to give Marie the ultimate test. It happened one afternoon when she and Len were in a hotel room, going through the preliminaries of lovemaking. Linda was nude, dancing with Len and moving her body against his. His erection was hard against her and his face was flushed. She lured him over to the bed, lay down, and, as he was getting on top of her, receded into my mind, leaving Marie in charge.

Marie was shocked to find herself in bed with Len. She pushed him back, rolling him off the bed. She sat up quickly and pulled the covers close around her. "My God, you were going to . . ."

"I was going to fuck you," said Len, his voice cold. He

was hurt and frustrated. His words came slowly, as though he was fighting for control.

"You're out of your mind, Linda. You know that? You're out of your fucking mind. I've been screwing you for weeks now. I've laid you under the truck, in motels, and even had you while leaning against a goddamned tree."

"Please . . . I need time to sort this all out."

"Now are we going to get it on together or aren't we?"

The incident was not the only time Marie found herself in bed with Len. Although Linda preferred having intercourse with Len, then letting Marie have the body, she began periodically having Marie take over just before intercourse. Each time the change in personality was obvious to Len. Gradually Marie accepted Len. She yielded and accepted this new dimension of her life even though it was against everything she had valued. It was just another part of the vast black holes that occupied so much of her memory.

Marie's relationship with Craig became increasingly strained. Although he never caught her with Len, Craig was certain Marie was having affairs. He began drinking heavily and made no pretense of affection for her.

Marie couldn't help comparing Len with Craig. Len was self-assured, well read, and almost Victorian in the way he felt a woman should be cared for. He sought a wild, uninhibited sex life but, away from the bedroom, Marie felt he was like the handsome hero of a romantic novel. By comparison, Craig seemed like a sniveling adolescent, selfish and uncaring. She moved out of the bedroom she shared with Craig, spending her nights on the couch.

Linda was delighted with Marie's change in attitude since it made her efforts so much easier. Finally, after four months of Marie sleeping on the couch, Linda took control and told Craig she was filing for divorce.

Craig was crushed by the divorce action, a divorce Marie learned about only after Linda had filed the papers. There was no love lost between himself and his wife but he looked upon the end of this marriage as a second failure in his life. He had lost the first woman he married and now it was happening again. Instead of accepting the fact that human relationships don't always work out, he thought of himself as the ultimate loser. He was certain he would be ridiculed at work for not being man enough to satisfy a woman.

The day Craig realized there would be no talking his wife out of a divorce, he decided to punish her.

The couple ate dinner in silence, then Marie gathered up the dishes and went into the kitchen to wash them. She returned to the living room when she was done.

"Craig?" said Marie, looking around the room. "Craig, where are you?"

There was no answer.

Marie wandered from room to room, looking for her husband. She even opened the bedroom closets, half suspecting he was hiding, playing some childish game to scare her. But there was no Craig. Then, as she started to leave the bedroom, she happened to glance out the window and noticed that the light inside the garage was turned on. Craig must have gone out there for some reason.

Marie walked out to the garage to see what her husband was doing. As she opened the door, she saw Craig, his head in a noose, the end of which was tied to one of the roof beams. His body was limp and still, his face blue. He was not struggling in any way.

Marie screamed and ran back to the house. Grabbing a sharp kitchen knife, she returned to the garage and quickly severed the rope holding Craig suspended above the ground.

Craig's body dropped, and Marie realized too late that she should have tried to absorb some of the shock of his fall. Instead, he struck the ground, his head bouncing against the rake.

Although close to death, Craig's body fought the trauma

it had endured. As Marie felt his neck, trying to tell if it was broken, she heard him begin to breathe. At first his chest seemed to convulse, the breathing sounding like short, snorting gasps. Then it came more naturally, and Marie began slapping his face, trying to rouse him to consciousness. When the breathing became even and regular, she raced to the telephone and called the only person she could think to ask for help—Len.

Len and his wife were quite concerned. They told Marie to call an ambulance on the chance that Craig still needed medical assistance. She did and, after the hospital made certain there was no permanent physical damage, Craig was transferred to the psychiatric ward for tests and treatment during the next three weeks.

I almost killed him, thought Marie. If I hadn't asked for a divorce, he never would have tried to kill himself. It's my fault. I might as well have tried to murder him in cold blood. I'm no good. I'm a rotten, worthless person who doesn't deserve to exist.

The more Marie observed her husband, the less guilty she felt. She realized that he was using her for his own ends.

Marie's guilt feelings were encouraged by Craig's co-workers. When he returned from the hospital, the doctor wanted him to have a long rest, so he was given a leave of absence from his job. The other employees knew the suicide attempt had occurred after Marie had asked for a divorce. Rather than trying to understand her feelings in the matter, they made Marie the villain. Linda had flirted with a number of them and her affair with Len was suspected by several.

Former friends of the couple ignored Marie or were abrupt when talking with her, letting her know they felt nothing but contempt for her having driven Craig to suicide. The fact that he was unstable and would have used almost any incident to act self-destructively didn't enter their minds.

They chose not to see Craig as emotionally disturbed but rather viewed Marie as an "almost" murderess.

Though Marie felt guilty, Linda wasn't about to let Craig's stunt keep her from Len.

Once Linda and Len were legally freed from their respective spouses, the two of them got married. Oddly, Linda chose to not go on the honeymoon, however. Apparently she wanted Marie to become completely adjusted to the new living situation with Len so she wouldn't have to worry about Marie's divorcing the only man about whom Linda ever cared. She let Marie go on the honeymoon, a trip Marie seemed to enjoy. When she returned, she fully accepted the new situation of being Len's wife.

7

PERSONALITY CONFLICTS

Len made a good living with the telephone company but his previous marriages had left him with expensive obligations. He had to pay $350 a month child support for his seven children. As a result, the only way Len and Marie could make ends meet was by her taking a job.

Marie delighted in the chance to have a job though it upset Len not to be able to support her completely from his earnings. She decided she wanted to try a new field, abandoning waitress and restaurant work entirely. She turned to the electronics field, enrolled in a course in the assembly of electronics equipment, received high marks, and obtained a job at a local plant. Each day she sat tightly packed with other workers on a bench on an assembly line, using her skills in what became a routine, monotonous task. Even worse was the feeling of claustrophobia she experienced, a sensation which caused her to spend lunch hours and breaks walking about outside the plant.

Marie never complained about her feelings and frustrations. Instead she concentrated on working as rapidly and efficiently as she could, receiving promotion after promotion for her efforts. She quickly rose to a supervisory position and received a "Top Secret" military clearance to work on defense contract projects destined for use in Vietnam. Linda was so bored with Marie's job that she never tried to take over at work.

The rapid promotions at the defense plant gave Marie a sense of self-worth. She could succeed at something. She had always been ashamed of her limited education in the past. However, she suddenly realized she could become anything she wanted to be if she just studied hard enough. She began thinking in terms of having a career.

Romantic novels had always appealed to Marie. She had a good imagination and fantasized herself in the role of the beautiful nurse who was adored by the handsome doctor as they labored side by side, saving lives. Even though she felt herself happily married to Len, the idea of being a part of the medical profession seemed very appealing. She convinced Len to let her quit her job and enroll in a school to learn to be a licensed vocational nurse.

During this period of time, Craig had remarried but he remained fond of Marie. Every few weeks he would go out drinking by himself and, when drunk, come over to see Len and Marie.

Craig talked of still being in love with Marie. He said she was the only person who ever won his heart.

Marie resented her ex-husband's actions, but Len had compassion for him. He felt that if it helped Craig to come by the house and cry on their shoulders, he was happy to listen to him.

Two weeks before Christmas, in 1971, Craig went on a drinking spree. Then he called Marie, his speech slurred by liquor. He talked about their life together, his many problems, and his new wife and the two children she had by a previous marriage. When he finished talking and weeping, he suddenly said, "Marie, are you happy with your new life?"

"Yes, Craig. Yes, I'm happy."

The next morning Len surprised Marie by showing up where she worked. "It's about Craig," he began, not certain how to tell her the news. "He put a gun to his head and shot himself."

Marie became hysterical. She rushed to the hospital to see him, but it was too late. He died before she could reach the intensive care unit.

Long after the funeral, long after Marie had come to accept the fact that Craig's suicide was the result of his emotional disturbance and not her actions, she still felt guilt. She was never able to escape the feeling that somehow, in some way, she might have prevented the tragic outcome of his life.

Nurse's training came as a shock to Marie. A student nurse assigned to the hospitals is often given the dirtiest, most unpleasant tasks possible. Instead of standing shoulder to shoulder with the doctor, Marie was carting bed pans and cleaning vomit.

The work assignments changed regularly and during one period of training, Marie was fortunate enough to be working in the medical ward of one of the country's finest private hospitals. The patients had more money than the ones in the public facilities, places which served indigent winos among others, and Marie thought the work might be easier. The atmosphere was warm and friendly, as most of the nurses were anxious to assist the students in learning the needed skills of the profession. However, one older nurse had nothing but contempt for the students and this included Marie.

It was 7 A.M. when the older nurse approached Marie and announced that she was to go to room 210 and assist the orderly with a patient. "What's wrong with him?" asked Marie.

"What difference does that make?" snapped the older nurse. "You students are supposed to do whatever is necessary to learn proper patient care. The patient in 210 needs help and the orderly can't handle him alone." A slight smile crossed her lips but Marie didn't notice the momentary change in expression.

Marie hurried down the corridor, opened the door to the room, and smiled at the man sitting on the bed. His hospital gown, never designed to provide properly modest coverage, was hiked up on his waist so the entire lower portion of his anatomy was exposed to view. Marie felt sorry for him, knowing how humiliating the lack of covering could be. "Good morning," she said warmly.

An orderly was standing by the patient, holding on to one arm. "Get the hell over on the other side of the bed and hang on to this guy," he snarled. There was no other greeting.

What sort of a bastard are you? thought Marie as she hurried to do what she was told. This patient is a human being with feelings that might easily be hurt. He shouldn't be treated like something that is a nuisance to the staff. He's our whole reason for having our jobs. She vowed she would say something to the orderly when they were alone together.

Marie walked over to the side, worked her shoulder under the man's arm, and held on to him. "I'll be right back," said the orderly, leaving the room.

"And how are you feeling today?" asked Marie. There was no response.

"My name is Marie Peters. I'm sorry I didn't get a chance to learn yours." Again there was no answer.

Slowly the man's body began to slip forward. Marie pushed against his downward momentum to try and keep him on the bed. "You're slipping," she said. "Perhaps if you hold on to me..." And then she got a closer look at the man. He was dead. She felt for his vital signs and realized that he might have been dead for quite some time. The bastard orderly had run out and left her with a corpse without once mentioning that fact to her.

A chill ran through Marie and her body shook involuntarily. She had never handled a dead person before and it was one aspect of nursing she never really expected to encounter. She was going to be the kind of nurse whose patients always improve under her care. She had no reason to ever consider that one of them might not live. And here she was trying to hold up a dead man whose body was slipping ever faster to the floor.

Marie stooped down, trying to use her body as a wedge to stop the corpse and return him to an upright position. She felt his weight against her and somehow managed to restore him to a balanced position. But the sensation of his lifeless body against her own wouldn't leave her skin even though he was no longer touching her. It was as though, in death, his contact would be permanent.

The orderly returned, pushing a gurney. It was a cart used for transporting patients around the hospital. The corpse was to be loaded on the cart, then covered in such a way that he looked like a living patient being wheeled to surgery. It was felt that other patients and their visitors should not be aware of a death in the hospital since it could be psychologically harmful. Every effort had to be made to keep the people who weren't on the staff from knowing that a patient had died.

Marie was in a state approaching shock. She forced herself to think of the task at hand, nothing more. She helped place the dead man on the gurney, covering his body with a sheet and wrapping his head as though he had just been in surgery. The corpse's face was yellow, the result of the cirrhosis of the liver that had taken his life. He had been a chronic alcoholic prior to his death and his face was as deeply rutted as a country road after a harsh winter's spring thaw.

Marie and the orderly moved the gurney swiftly toward the elevator, then rode to the basement where there was a "cold room" for bodies waiting transportation to the mortuary. Marie stared at the dead man as she moved, wondering who he was and who he left behind. Alcoholics have no friends but the bottle. Who would mourn the loss of an apparently wasted life?

At last the body was deposited in the cold room, the door

closed, and the assignment completed. Marie leaned against the wall, tears coming to her eyes. Her body shook involuntarily and she knew she was becoming hysterical.

It had all been so cold. In the books she read, people never died like that. A passing was always a quiet affair with the family and friends gathered about the person who had lived a full and useful life. It was a time of mutual comforting and, though the end was near, there was always hope in everyone's heart.

This death had been as cold and impersonal as the farm slaughter of cattle bred for market. The dead man was treated like a piece of meat to be pushed and carted and abandoned. Was this what nursing was really all about? Did you have to become cold and unfeeling in order to be a success? Was the attitude of the nurse who had given her the assignment the one she should have—insensitive and unthinking?

A senior nurse, who was also an instructor, happened by after the corpse had been put away. She put her arm around Marie and led her to the nurses' lounge, a place that was normally "off limits" to lowly students. There Marie told her what had happened; the instructor was outraged. She said the nurse who had given Marie the assignment had behaved inexcusably. Marie should have been better prepared, at least so far as being told that the patient had died.

Marie felt better after the talk. She also came to the conclusion that she wanted to try and help men like the one who had died in that room. Alcoholics were life's losers in the eyes of most doctors and nurses. No one wanted to deal with an individual whose body might be covered with shit and vomit and urine. No one wanted to work with somebody who they cleaned up, dried out, and sent off sober only to have him return drunk, vomiting, and out of his head with delirium tremens. Such people were despised in life and dumped like rotten meat when they died. The only way such people would ever really have a chance in life would be if someone in the profession started to care about them. Marie was determined to be such a person.

Marie's determination to become a top nurse proved far stronger than Linda's desire to go drinking, dancing, and whoring, so Linda seldom took control. Marie's waking hours were spent in intense concentration. In addition to the class work, she went to the library during her free time and read every book she could find that related to what she was trying to learn.

The hospital activities with which Marie was involved were specially planned to coordinate with her classroom instruction. While Marie was listening to lectures on communicable diseases, she worked in the tuberculosis ward of the county hospital. When she studied the heart and respiratory system, she worked with patients suffering from heart disease, emphysema, and similar ailments. And when she studied psychology, she worked in the psychiatric ward, the geriatric unit, and the alcoholic detoxification unit.

When she worked with the psychiatric patients, she empathized with their suffering. Many had made the ultimate adjustment. They had found peace in the institutional setting and would never function well in the outside world.

I'm not like that, thought Marie. There can't be too much wrong with me if I'm able to perform nursing duties and care for others. Even my drinking isn't bad. I get to work every day and, aside from an occasional hangover or memory loss, I really have few problems. I guess you have to work in a place like this for a while to gain a proper perspective on yourself. I'm going to just apply myself and stop worrying about the state of my mind. Obviously I'm coping with life very well.

Marie graduated from nurse's training and immediately found a job in a private hospital specializing in the care of alcoholics. The hospital was run by Dr. Don Lamont, a man Marie felt typified the best of the medical professional. He was tall, with dark, wavy hair and the kind of face that made him look like he had been selected from a Hollywood movie studio's central casting department. He ran the hospital in addition to having a private practice. Each patient paid at least $40 a day to stay there, and additional expenses invariably sent their bills soaring. Dr. Lamont, himself, received $8 for every visit which, as Marie later learned, meant the two or three minutes he spent with a patient while making his rounds. The regular care was provided by the nursing staff.

The longer Marie worked at the hospital, the more she learned about Dr. Lamont. He was married to a woman who worked as a hospital secretary but he had at least one ex-wife and some children in his past. His alimony payments were high, but his expensive fees enabled him to live in one of the more exclusive sections of the city and to take annual vacations in Europe.

Marie looked upon Dr. Lamont as a noble, self-sacrificing individual, despite evidence to the contrary which was recognized by everyone but Marie. She felt his valuable time shouldn't have to be spent with minor details of the patients' care. She began handling record keeping and other detail work she had seen the doctor doing from time to time. He was delighted with her interest and began making considerable effort to get to know her.

It was during this period that Marie decided she wanted even more training than she had already received. She made the decision to return to school, this time to earn a full college degree as a registered nurse. But her full-time work schedule, which started at seven in the morning, and her part-time class schedule meant that she was able to get very little sleep.

"Are you still trying to go twenty-four hours a day without sleeping?" asked Dr. Lamont.

Marie smiled. "If I'm going to get my degree, it's the only way I can do it. I promise I won't let it interfere with my work, though."

"Don't worry about that. You're the best nurse we've got.

I just thought you might like something to help you stay alert during the day."

And with that, Marie was introduced to pep pills—"uppers" as they are called. Dr. Lamont prescribed amphetamines to keep her body racing all day and evening. Later he added a prescription for "downers" so she could relax enough to sleep the few hours available to her.

Marie had studied the effects of different medications while in school and knew how dangerous the drugs she was taking could be. But Marie was operating on both an intellectual and an emotional level at that point. Her mind told her the drugs were dangerous but her heart told her the doctor was only concerned with her best interests. She couldn't imagine why a doctor would give her the prescription, a prescription she could have refilled as often as she liked, if there was any danger for her.

During this time Linda had been fairly inactive. There were few amnesia periods for Marie, her concentration on nursing studies apparently being strong enough to keep Linda from taking over with any frequency. However, every few weeks Linda would regain control and go out seeking excitement.

Len was bitter about Marie's nursing career. He had approved her going to school but that was when he thought it wouldn't take much of her time. He never realized how important a part of her life the pursuit of the RN degree would prove to be. He was jealous of the time she spent at the hospital and at the area college. He began fighting with her almost daily and constantly pressured her to tell him where she was going each time she left home.

One night, when Marie was on her way home, she felt nauseated and dizzy. She started to pull her car to the side of the road as her body slumped forward, then jerked erect. Linda was in control.

Linda glanced in the rear-view mirror, adjusting the wig on her head. Both Linda and Marie liked wigs, though Linda preferred more daring styles than Marie wore. Whenever she had control, Linda liked to shop for new wigs, putting them in the closet where Marie wouldn't discover them easily. Occasionally Marie would return them when she found them, shocked by the thought that she might have bought something styled in such a fashion. At other times she just left them on the shelf, not understanding how they got there, yet not willing to deal with it.

I need some excitement, thought Linda, pulling into a bowling alley a few hundred yards from where she had taken control.

She picked up a man and spent some time with him. They had been drinking and dancing in several nightspots and both were feeling relaxed. As they pulled into the lot, the man was about to suggest they spend the rest of the night together when Linda spotted Len.

"So there you are, you slut!" said Len, a rifle cradled in his arms. He had been cruising the city looking for her. It was by chance that he spotted Marie's car in the lot. "Get in my car!"

The son of a bitch is really pissed this time, thought Linda, doing as she was told. No sense messing with a hothead carrying a rifle.

After several minutes of driving, Len turned off onto a dirt road, drove a short way along the path, and then said, "Out, bitch!"

Linda grabbed Len's wrist, pulled it to her mouth, and bit down hard, drawing blood from the wound. He jerked it away, opened the car door, and half fell from the vehicle.

Linda leaped from her door, ran around to Len, and stomped on his foot. He slapped her face, then doubled over as she slammed her knee into his groin. She began striking him with her feet, knees, and hands, using all the force her rage could trigger. Len's face was bleeding, his nose seemed broken, and he was having trouble breathing by the time she finished. He fell across the car, rolled his body toward the door, and managed to drop half onto the back seat, half onto the floor of the car.

I must be overtired, thought Marie, looking about the house. The last thing I remember is being in the car, driving home. I must have made the trip in my sleep. Maybe those pills I've been taking have gotten the best of me. I certainly don't remember coming home.

"Len? Where are you?" Marie began walking from room to room.

"Marie..." The voice was faint and followed by the sound of someone coughing and choking. It was coming from the side door. She turned and saw her husband, barely conscious, leaning against the frame.

"Leonard!" she exclaimed, her face horrified. "My God, honey, what happened to you?" She rushed to him, putting her body underneath his so she could support his weight while helping him to the couch. "Were you in a fight? Were you mugged? Oh, my poor darling. What happened?"

Leonard was shocked by his wife's reaction. "You... You... You beat me..." he whispered. "On that back road. You..."

Marie was only half listening. With her trained eyes and hands she was carefully examining her husband for physical damage. Some of his ribs seemed broken and she knew there were probably internal injuries. She helped him back to the car and drove him to the hospital where her suspicions were confirmed. He had several broken ribs. He was carefully bandaged, then released in her care.

On the way home Len repeated what had happened.

Maybe I should tell him the truth, thought Marie. Maybe

I should tell him I don't remember hurting him.

No, I can't do that. He either won't believe me or he's liable to leave me. I need Len. I need what support I get from him. I'm not ready to be on my own right now.

There was little time for Marie to worry about her husband. Events were occurring at work that would shortly overwhelm her.

Dr. Lamont had become increasingly friendly with Marie, often touching her when they were where his wife couldn't see them. Marie took the touching as a gesture of friendship, never imagining that the doctor, whom she idolized, might have something more in mind.

It was raining the day it happened. An elderly alcoholic was suffering from severe dehydration while undergoing withdrawal. Marie knew he needed liquids and she wanted to start some fluid intravenously—directly into the bloodstream since there was no way the extremely sick man could swallow at that time. But an I.V. could not be given without a doctor's permission. Since he wasn't close at hand, Marie telephoned him to explain what was happening.

Marie was surprised to find herself sexually aroused by the doctor when he came rushing into the dehydrated patient's room.

Dr. Lamont seemed to sense Marie's feelings as he worked. As soon as the crisis had passed, he took Marie into the next room.

It was like a fantasy for Marie, a fantasy in real life. Suddenly she was the nurse in all those romantic novels and Dr. Lamont was her hero. For the first time, Marie was responding to a man rather than being cajoled after finding herself in bed with a stranger. She was prepared to let herself go.

Marie started to kiss the doctor again, but he put his hands on her shoulders and gently but firmly pushed down. He wanted her on her knees.

Marie felt as though she might vomit. Her stomach ached

as she struggled in her mind to cope with the knowledge that Dr. Lamont, her idol, wanted her to do something she felt was perverted. Her head felt as though it was spinning and she seemed to be caught in a bottomless whirlpool.

So the great god Lamont is just another son of a bitch who likes having his cock sucked, thought Linda. Shit, I don't know why the hell she's so surprised. Men have been using her for years. What difference does it make how they do it?

Linda looked up at the doctor and smiled. It doesn't matter if the bastard's a doctor or a laborer. They're all animals. Well, what the hell.

No sense disappointing the supplier of good times. You can't have a happy hour without the pills. If sucking his cock will keep the prescriptions coming, it's the least I can do. She lowered her head and proceeded to give Dr. Lamont the pleasure Marie found too disgusting to contemplate.

She was rewarded. The doctor gave Marie a wider variety of drugs and never questioned why she used so many.

Since the relationship between Linda and the doctor became a regular one, Lamont felt his wife would become suspicious of Linda's frequent visits to the private office. The doctor pretended Linda was seeing him as a patient rather than just an employee. He set up a phony chart which indicated Linda was receiving regular "treatment." After each visit, Marie was sent a bill for the doctor's normal fee. Because Marie had no knowledge or memory of what went on during those visits, she assumed the doctor really was treating her for some physical problem. She always paid the bills.

The widely varying experiences of the radically different women who alternated in controlling my body over the years seem rather strange at first, but the difference between a healthy mind and the mind of someone suffering from multiple personality is not all that great.

Multiple personality is actually a form of what doctors call dissociation, as I learned while in therapy. Dissociation, in a mild form, is experienced by everyone during their lives.

A form of normal dissociation occurs when someone talks in his or her sleep. Somewhat less common is the sleepwalker, yet even this type of dissociating individual is seldom mentally ill.

Everyone can be said to have different sides to their personalities. In the bedroom you might be a sexually aggressive lover. When vacationing at the beach you might be childlike and frolicsome. And in the office you might be sober and hard-working. Yet because you are normal, these behavior patterns are blended into a whole, "integrated" personality. Your behavior matches your circumstances and is always appropriate to what is going on. In the case of a multiple personality, each aspect of the personality becomes rigid and independent.

There are a number of factors which are known to contribute to multiple personality, all of which I experienced as a child. A feeling of being unwanted is a part of the problem, as is the creation of an imaginary playmate who becomes a "real" person in the child's mind. Child abuse is usually experienced.

Leonard was the first person to recognize Marie's problem, though he had no idea she was a multiple personality.

The situation with Dr. Lamont became less and less tolerable for Marie. She had no idea that Linda was having a sexual affair with him, but she did sense that something was wrong with their relationship. She felt it would be best if she looked for work elsewhere, a change which greatly upset Linda, who didn't want to give up the drugs Dr. Lamont was prescribing.

Before Marie could quit working at the hospital, Linda decided she would "kill" Marie.

Linda located one of Marie's uniforms, put it on, and went to the alcoholic treatment center.

She went straight to the locked medicine storage case, found a bottle of Methaqualone, and placed it in her purse. The medication was one of the strongest prescription sleeping tablets available and thus one of the most dangerous. It was always kept locked in a limited-access medicine safe.

Linda returned home, went into the bedroom, and locked the door. She opened the bottle of Methaqualone and swallowed the entire contents—thirty tablets. But nothing happened. She reached into a package purchased that afternoon and removed a holder of highly polished, double-edged blades.

Most multiple personality cases have an alter-personality who is filled with rage and a potential for violence. Sometimes this person lashes out against others. She or he might beat up strangers in bars or family members who criticize their behavior.

At other times, as was the case with Linda, the alter-personality becomes self-destructive. Linda looked upon Marie as an enemy. Marie had respect, an important position, and pride in what she did. In effect, I had grown to hate a part of myself.

Linda touched the blade to her skin. The bedroom door handle turned back and forth several times. Len had returned home early. It didn't matter, though. Even if he got through the heavy lock, she had wedged the big double bed, hardwood chest of drawers, and the rest of the furniture flush against the door. The furniture was so heavy and carefully positioned that it would be impossible for one man to break through.

"Marie? Open this door, Marie!" shouted Len, pounding against it. "I want to talk with you!"

Linda didn't answer. She was concentrating on lacerating her arm. The blood flowed rapidly, making her work more difficult. Several times she wiped her arm against her blouse so she could clear enough blood to see where she had cut and where she had yet to slash. By the time she heard the sirens in the distance, she had made a dozen incisions in her arm.

"Mrs. Peters?" It was a new voice—male—deeper than Len's. "We're police officers, Mrs. Peters. We're here to help you."

"Then go away!" shouted Linda. "Leave me alone." The sleeping pills should have been working faster than they were. She wasn't tired. In fact, she was excited. Her adrenaline was flowing rapidly. She was high, feeling a little like when she was drunk. She watched the blood flowing relentlessly from her body, yet had no sensation of impending death.

There was a pounding against the door. It was light at first, then harder and more rhythmic. The policemen were using their shoulders to batter the door. Their bodies struck together so their combined weight would have more impact. It was slow work, but gradually the wood around the lock splintered and split apart. A few minutes more and they managed to push the furniture far enough back to squeeze inside.

The first police officer started toward Linda who was standing near the bathroom. Her clothing was soaked with blood and it seemed obvious to the officer that she was in no condition to put up a fight. He extended his hand to her and said, "Don't be frightened, Mrs. Peters. We're here to help you."

Linda stepped toward the police officer, then suddenly brought her fist up and struck him on the jaw. He was well over six feet tall, lean and muscular. He had been in the Marine Corps and was more than able to hold his own in barroom brawls. He thought he could handle anything—until that moment. When the blow landed, his eyes glazed over and his unconscious body dropped, striking the dresser, rolling against the bed and onto the floor.

A second police officer started toward Linda. She bent her knee, then sent her foot sharply forward, viciously striking him in the groin. His body doubled over into a fetal position, his eyes tightly closed. Sweat suddenly poured from his face and a low moan rose from his lips.

"Pigs!" screamed Linda, as the remaining four officers moved warily into the room, keeping their distance while attempting to surround her. "Goddamned pigs!"

Linda's body tensed. Her shoulders were slightly hunched and she was carefully balanced on her feet, ready to spring at whichever police officer dared to get too close. She was oblivious to the blood loss, a loss so severe it should have sent her body into shock. The rage that made her try to take her own life was now foscused on the men who were attempting to be her rescuers. She was going to kill them—one by one or all at once, however they dared approach her.

Suddenly the police officers lunged. They moved at the same time, preventing Linda from isolating anyone for punishment. Two men grabbed her arms and the other two went for her legs, hoping to stop her wild thrashing.

Linda, her left arm almost useless, fought with an intensity that few men could have matched. Her nails clawed the face of one officer and she bit the ear of another. She tugged at the hair of a third and butted her head against the nose of the fourth. Two ambulance attendants and Len watched helplessly. There was no way they could work themselves into the ceaselessly moving tangle of bodies and flailing arms and legs in order to aid in subduing her.

Finally one of the officers managed to wrench Linda's right arm behind her back. He snapped a handcuff on her wrist, attaching it to her left hand when that arm was also forced behind her. He knew the cuffs might injure her, but it seemed the only way to get her to the emergency room at the hospital. Then the police officers, their uniforms torn, their faces bloody, tightly gripped Linda's legs and shoulders and carried her out to the stretcher.

The fight wasn't over for Linda, though. She was strapped

to the stretcher, her legs and arms immobilized after the police, carefully gripping her, had removed the handcuffs. Additional restraints went across her chest and around her waist. Yet Linda continued thrashing her head back and forth, striking the ambulance attendants who were working desperately to cover her wounds and keep her alive while they transported her to the hospital.

The emergency room staff was waiting for Linda but they had no idea what they were going to encounter. She was wheeled into the room on a stretcher, her eyes closed, her breathing shallow, her body still. It seemed as though the blood loss and Methaqualone overdose had rendered her unconscious. The restraints were removed and she was placed on an operating table where the doctors and nurses could tend to her wounds and pump the drug from her stomach.

"Bastards!" shouted Linda, opening her eyes and glaring at the surprised hospital staff. One doctor was holding a suture, ready to begin stitching one of her wounds. She knocked his arm aside, sending his instruments flying across the room.

A nurse reached for Linda's left arm, only to be stopped by a hard punch to her stomach. She doubled over, trying desperately not to retch. The battle had begun again.

Fortunately for the doctors, Linda was weaker than when the police tangled with her at home. She was quickly subdued, then lost consciousness, giving the staff the opportunity they needed to repair the damage she had done to her body. She didn't awaken again until she was bandaged and under close observation in the psychiatric ward.

The official admission forms showed that Linda was suffering from depression. She was expected to see a psychiarist during her stay, but she didn't know any. Linda asked one of the nursing staff who she would recommend.

"Why don't you talk with Dr. Brewster?" suggested the nurse. She pointed to a man at the far end of the hall.

That is the most pompous asshole I've ever seen in my life, thought Linda. Look at the way he's strutting down the hall, flaunting his title of Shrink like it was a golden banner. He's moving like a rooster in a hen house. Hell, that's what he is—Brewster the rooster!

Or maybe he's a bear, thought Linda, when the doctor came closer. She could see he was a large man, well over six feet tall, and he must have weighed at least 225 pounds. His clothing was rumpled and he had a heavy growth of beard, the result of spending the night with an emergency patient. Linda decided he looked like an owl who'd been spending hours chasing a mouse and the mouse got away.

Linda's attempt to kill Marie, my attempt to take my own life, was, like all such acts, a cry for help. But the personalities were still too busy raging at each other to begin to try and pull themselves together to form one whole person.

So when Linda first met Dr. Brewster while recovering, she was far from ready to reach out to him for help. Linda was concerned only with trying to manipulate him for the help she thought she needed.

"You asked to see me?" said Dr. Brewster. He smiled at Linda, revealing a gap between two of his front teeth.

If this is the best shrink they can give you around here, Lord help the sickies. "Yes, doctor," she said quietly. "I don't have a psychiatrist and I wonder if you could take my case."

Play it cool, thought Linda. Give the creep a tale of woe and see what drugs he'll prescribe. Hell, staying here could be a real trip if this guy cooperates.

But the doctor didn't cooperate. He prescribed a mild pain killer and gave strict orders that the dosage was to be constantly reduced during the next few days as Linda's wounds began to heal. Then she was to be taken off all medication, regardless of the type.

Linda was angered by the way she was treated and refused to cooperate fully. She attended a number of therapy sessions, saying whatever she thought might get her released, refusing to listen to anything that was suggested to her. After several days she was considered well enough to leave.

8

LOCKED UP INSIDE

Marie wanted to forget the suicide attempt. As a nurse, her job was to give comfort and help to the living. It was an embarrassment to be constantly reminded of the disrespect she had shown her own life when she slashed her wrists. Yet the partial paralysis she had caused in her left wrist kept her keenly aware of a problem that would not go away. The suicide attempt also cost Marie her job at the alcohol treatment facility.

Dr. Lamont had been at the hospital when Linda was brought in for treatment. He read her chart and realized she was emotionally unstable. He didn't know what might have driven her to suicide and he didn't care. Nor was he worried about what might happen to the patients in her charge. However, an emotionally distraught woman just might tell his wife about the affair he had been having and he didn't want to risk that. Some other nurse could be found to satisfy his desire for oral sex.

The year was 1972 and Marie found a job working for the Public Health Department as the first nurse ever employed to work full time at the county jail. She was given preliminary special training in a free clinic in Watsonville, California, an agricultural area where migrant workers were in need of information on family planning as well as other aspects of health care. When Marie went to the jail, she was to provide the female inmates with both testing services and special care relating to their gynecologic needs.

Marie had a unique role in the county jail system in

that she was an independent individual who had no concern with the punitive aspects of inmate care. For example, she refused to conduct searches for the narcotics which were routinely hidden in all body openings by desperate addicts. But she wouldn't leave the addicts' sides if they were in the throes of withdrawal. She didn't care if the inmates were guilty or innocent, dangerous or passive. She was going to give them the care and medical counseling they needed, regardless of their circumstances.

This is the kind of work I should have been doing all along, thought Marie, as she busied herself giving Pap smears, pelvic examinations, and other tests meant to spot the early symptoms of numerous diseases. I'm doing something worthwhile with my time and there's no chance to feel sorry for myself. I don't feel the need to drink and I'm not having those periods of lost time. There was nothing wrong with my mind except that it was inactive. I don't know why I tried to slash my wrists, but that's all behind me. This is a place where I am truly needed and I'm going to dedicate myself to it.

Marie's biggest shock during her early days in the jail came the morning she arrived, walked to Holding Tank #3, and saw her brother, Al, among the inmates. He and his wife had had an argument the previous night, during which he had lost his temper and beat her mercilessly, though neighbors fortunately called the police before he could kill her. When he heard the sirens, he raced from his house to where his motorcycle was parked, leaped on it, and accelerated down the street. The police gave chase, catching him when he lost control while going over an embankment. He was charged with "felony wife beating" among other things and had to be treated for a broken leg and numerous cuts that required a total of seventy-five stitches. He eventually served three months in the county jail.

Linda had nothing but contempt for Al. Every time she

saw him, she remembered the incestuous relations of their childhood and the rape when she was in her early teens. But Marie had no such memories. She and Al had never been very close and she had frequently been hurt by his taunts when they were children. Yet Marie remained filled with compassion for his plight, regardless of his crime.

Marie knew the nightmare world of the jail and did what she could to help her brother through the period he would have to stay there. She gave him a slightly stronger than normal dose of sleeping medication when he wanted it so he wouldn't have to hear the screams of the addicts, the retching of the drunks, and the other night sounds of the jail. She also saw to it that he had cigarettes and money for candy, though technically such acts of kindness on her part were illegal. In fact, one time Marie ordered Al to the nursing office on the pretext of having to check the cast on his leg. While he was there, unseen by the jailer outside, she treated him to a McDonald's cheeseburger she had sneaked inside.

I've always known there was something wrong with Marie's mind, but I think she's gone completely bananas. My God, working all day with those stinking addicts and muggers and drunks . . . It makes my flesh crawl to know this body has been in and out of all those cells.

And the hours she keeps. When I do get control of the body, I'm physically drained. If she's got to be out doing something all day, why can't it be drinking or getting laid or something else that would be constructive?

Some of those guards are pretty cute, I've got to admit. And the way they keep trying to touch her, I know they'd give anything to get inside her pants. Hell, don't they know she's not the type? What I ought to do is go in there for her and see if they're as good in bed as they claim.

Linda was nervous about going in the jail the first time she took control of Marie's body at work. She wasn't afraid of being attacked. She just hated the smells and sounds that seemed to overwhelm even those who didn't have to stay in the cells. However, she relaxed when she was able to make a date with a deputy sheriff named Pete. He was working as a jailer because the sheriff felt he was too violent to patrol the streets. Linda hoped that violence might make him more sexually exciting.

Linda took control of the body at the end of Marie's work shift. She drove home and immediately picked a fight with Len. She knew exactly what to say to enrage him and, when he was shouting and carrying on almost to the point of violence, she stalked out of the house. Len, disgusted with his wife, didn't follow, a fact on which Linda had been counting. She went immediately to the rendezvous.

Pete and Linda sat at the bar, drinking steadily, until Linda became bored. "I know a good motel," said Pete.

"All right, but I'm paying for the room," said Linda. Pete was surprised but wasn't about to argue. Anything that got him into bed with her was fine with him.

Linda insisted on paying because she felt it would give her control. To her way of thinking, whoever paid for the room dominated the sex act that followed. She would be using Pete for her gratification instead of his using her.

Pete and Linda each got in their cars, Pete taking the lead. Then, without warning Linda accelerated, passed Pete, and led him to the sleaziest hotel she could find. The room only cost $6, but, after intercourse, Linda came to the conclusion that even that price was too high for what she had gotten.

"Baby, you're the greatest thing since the invention of the wheel," said Pete, leaning back in bed, a smile on his face.

Linda grunted in acknowledgment. The son of a bitch would have said that if I lay there unconscious with a bag over my head, she thought to herself. Every time I get plastered with some guy before we jump into bed, the animal says I'm the greatest fuck he's ever had.

Despite Linda's dislike for Pete's "performance," she agreed to see him frequently. He was different from Len and she liked the variety. What she didn't like was having to sneak around all the time. The only answer was to divorce Len and regain her freedom.

Pete and Linda's dates began changing in ways Linda failed to recognize as potentially dangerous. He was increasingly rough during supposed moments of tenderness.

At first Linda thought Pete's actions were the result of an overwhelming animal passion. However, one day, as they were preparing for bed, he asked her if she was into pain. He wanted to have a sadomasochistic relationship with her.

"Hell, why not?" said Linda. I've tried everything else and it all ends up the same way, she thought. Besides, if it gets too bad, I can give the body back to Marie and really freak her out. She doesn't know anything about the affair, other than Pete's always mentioning our "good times." She probably thinks it's a line. I'd love to see what she does if I let her have the body when he's on me.

Pete began this new phase of their relationship gradually, slapping Linda on the face and arms. But as he beat her, he seemed to get more pleasure than he did from their intercourse. He became quite violent, scaring Linda and making her body ache. None of her bones were broken but she was bruised all over.

"You're mine now, bitch!" said Pete. "You hear me? I catch you so much as talking to someone else at the jail, I'm going to kick your ass. You understand?"

"Yes . . ." said Linda weakly.

Then, to emphasize his point, Pete hit Linda in the face and shoved her to the floor. He was wearing his boots and he put one foot heavily on her chest, saying, "I'll slice out your snatch if I catch you with someone else." Then he left.

Linda's hand was shaking as she lit a cigarette and tried

to smoke to calm her nerves. She was just beginning to relax when the phone rang. It was Pete who had been gone less than ten minutes. "You get your ass over to my house at ten tomorrow morning," he shouted.

"Okay," said Linda, annoyed and somewhat frightened. "Okay."

Both Pete and Marie were expected to be at work at seven the next morning. Thus Pete's request seemed odd to her but she decided to go along with it. She let Marie report to work as usual, then planned to take control long enough to go to Pete's house. She thought he was just nuts enough to kill her if she crossed him and that was something she wanted to avoid. If the body was going to meet with a violent end, she wanted it within her control. She would use pills, booze, and razor blades. She wasn't going to be beaten to death by a psychopathic madman in a deputy sheriff's uniform.

Linda left work, telling the jailers she had a meeting over at the Health Department, three miles away. She drove to Pete's house and went inside. He was married, but his wife, a teller at the local bank, was working.

Pete wanted one thing from Linda. He took her arm, dragged her into the bedroom, and made certain she saw his loaded revolver and handcuffs on a table by the bed. He started to undress, then told Linda to do the same.

When Linda was naked, Pete grabbed the handcuffs and used them to fasten her to a corner of the bed. He climbed on top of her and began fondling her body. Then, just before he reached a climax, Pete took his gun, held it to her head, and ordered her to say: "I love to fuck you, Pete." She did. She would have said anything he wanted at that moment.

And then it was over. For some reason, that morning's escapade was the last time Pete tried to have sex with Linda, or anything else to do with her. She stopped speaking to him and he apparently feared she might bring an assault charge against him if he wasn't careful. He had already been charged with beating some prisoners in the jail and he may have felt that a complaint by a Public Health Service nurse would result in his conviction. He didn't realize that his bedmate "victim" and the jail nurse were two different people with only a body in common.

Marie knew nothing of the divorce proceedings which Linda had begun until Len told her of them. She was shocked, genuinely amazed that not only was such an action taking place, but also that she apparently had a part in it.

At the same time, Marie had the feeling that divorce was the right action to take. She had an uneasy sense that something was happening to her. She was changing in subtle ways, as though in preparation for an event of major importance in her life.

Whatever Marie had to face, she knew she had to face it alone. Neither Len nor Tina could help her. Caring for them only added to the daily pressures she experienced. Divorce seemed an important step, though to what end, she did not know. Pete served to give her an out.

Marie seemed to mature during her time at the county jail. She saw a side of humanity she never knew existed, including the doctors. She realized how varied human beings could be, even within the medical profession.

During the period Marie held the job of county jail nurse, Linda was limited in the time she gained control. However, she was growing increasingly cautious. Linda also had the vague feeling of uneasiness about the future that Marie was experiencing. But to Linda, who knew of the other alter-personalities, the logical explanation was that Marie was going to take control full time.

Linda had already seen that Marie could control the body when she was dedicated to some project. When Marie received her nurse's training, for example, Linda almost never was able to do what she wanted. Linda increasingly felt the need to dominate. We were building toward a personality clash—but, unlike those conflicts that take place within families or on the job, mine was between personalities that lived in the same skin.

On the last day Marie worked at the county jail, Linda found the opening she'd been waiting for.

She grabbed glutethimide, a strong sleeping medicine, and chloral hydrate, the so-called knockout drops. Then, after dinner with Len that evening, Linda went to the bedroom and swallowed thirty-two ounces of the knockout drops and thirty tablets of the sleeping medication.

Three days after taking the drugs, Linda awakened in the county psychiatric hospital. Len had found her unconscious and managed to get help for her before it was too late.

County psychiatric hospitals are among the worst of the short-term care facilities for mental patients. It is where you go when you are too poor to afford treatment without tax support. When the police find a wino wandering the streets, out of his mind, they bring him to the county facility. When a little old lady is found eating out of garbage cans and talking to lamp posts, she also is brought to the county facility.

The county hospital has changed since I was there. It now has open, sunlit rooms, and a real effort is being made to make the facility livable for the patients. But such humane attitudes did not exist when I was spending time in such institutions—almost half of my adult life.

The hospital ward in which Linda was placed after over-dosing on medication consisted of small, cramped, almost dungeonlike rooms. The whores, winos, dope addicts, degenerates, and other low-lifes who had flipped out of their heads for one reason or another lived in quarters so close that it created added tension for everyone.

My alter-personalities were in the mental wards so frequently that it hardly seems possible it took so long for me to get well. Unfortunately the hospitals I entered were seldom equipped for therapy of genuine value. Many times a poorly trained staff, frustrated by the failures of whatever treatments were being tried, turned to radical methods of trying to restore sanity to the patients. For example, one therapist decided that we patients would benefit by releasing pent-up emotions. He had several patients sit around on the floor, howling like dogs. Everyone had a grand time acting like hounds baying at the moon, but what relationship that had to the underlying problems which had brought us to the hospital no one ever knew.

Some of the group sessions were handled by psychiatric social workers. In theory, a group therapy session involves people who can relate to one another and their problems. Rational discussion is carried on to try and get everyone to view themselves and the world in a more rational manner. The reality of such therapy was quite different.

The psychiatric social workers I encountered were not on salary for their group therapy sessions. Instead they were paid "piece rate." They received a set amount of money for each person in a particular group. Thus it was to their economic interest to bring as many patients to these group sessions as possible, regardless of whether or not this approach would benefit the patient.

One typical group included several people who were catatonic—unable to speak or relate to others. They sat looking vacantly ahead, never talking, never giving any indication they heard or understood what was going on around them. Others were so senile that they babbled quietly to themselves about events that had happened many years earlier—if they had occurred at all. One extremely obese woman spent the entire time playing solitaire, a game she pursued everywhere she went. A man brought in by the police proceeded to pull down his pants and masturbate in front of the group. A girl in her late teens or early twenties thought she had taken a trip to outer space after overdosing on a drug from which she never came down.

The psychiatric social worker who conducted the group was more like a circus ringmaster. Nothing of value was ever discussed because one or another of the extremely ill mental patients would keep "flipping out."

During all the years I was in and out of mental wards, almost no effort was made to get to understand me as an individual. Group therapy leaders played games with everyone. The sessions I had on a one-to-one basis were generally brief and meant to serve a preconceived notion. (For example, I was evaluated by both Dr. Brewster, well before I went to him in a genuine effort to get help, and other psychiatrists at the request of the courts. They wrote observations based on an interview and some brief testing, all of which were superficial. The law allows only a limited amount of time and money for these court-ordered tests, so this was the fault of the "system" rather than the doctors. If they had spent more time with me, perhaps they would have uncovered my problem much sooner.)

At other times a social worker was trying to prove a point that was also preconceived. For example, I was in jail for drunkenness when a social worker evaluated me. She felt all alcoholics were unfit mothers and she was there for the express purpose of taking Tina from me. Every question she asked was aimed at getting a response that would help her prove Tina should be removed from the home. She was uninterested in why I drank, whether or not I had ever abused Tina in any way, or if it was possible for me to get better. She never mentioned Alcoholics Anonymous or any other group which might have benefited me. She wanted Tina out of the family home and couldn't care less about my problems.

And so I went through the system year in and year out. Each "professional" I encountered was hung up on his or her own problems and beliefs. It was only by chance that I finally turned to someone who really cared about my future. And that was still one major crisis away.

9
COMING APART

It was bad enough that Linda, as an adult, was both an alcoholic and a drug addict. When she was in the hospital for the overdose described in the previous chapter, she even went so far as to steal bottles of mouthwash from the other patients. Many of these contained as much as 14 percent alcohol, so she could get a kick by drinking all the mouthwash she could get her hands on.

Looking back at those days with the perspective of someone who is finally whole, I keep wondering if Linda was trying to kill herself or save me. Perhaps she wasn't as tough as she appeared.

My problems were compounded when Linda decided to turn to crime to get some thrills. She had been feeling restless. She was sick of Len and the idea that she was burdened by Marie's family. She hated being around Tina and decided she needed to take drastic action if she was ever going to make her life change for the better.

Look at the little brat, thought Linda, watching Tina sitting on the living room floor. She was enjoying a cartoon show on television, laughing at the antics of the characters. How the hell can you go anywhere when you've always got to think of the kid. I've got to do something to get rid of the little brat.

The pills.

Linda went to the bathroom, opened the medicine chest, and removed seven pills.

"Tina, honey, I've got some candy for you."

Tina took the pills, popped one in her mouth and began sucking it. Suddenly she grimaced and said, "This candy tastes bad."

"Eat it anyway," said Linda, her voice becoming slightly harsh. She was nervous about the kid's not taking any. She had to kill her now. There might not be a chance later. Tina obediently swallowed the pills.

Linda watched Tina as the pills began to take effect. She could tell the child was having trouble keeping awake as she watched the set. There was nothing to do but wait.

Tina stretched out on the floor, lying on her stomach, her head turned sideways so it was against the carpet as she watched the set. Her vision had become blurred and she was giggling hysterically at the picture on the screen.

"What's so funny, Tina, honey?" asked Marie. She always enjoyed sharing the things that made her daughter happy. This was a very special daughter for her and she delighted in being a part of her childhood world.

"Those cats dancing on the television."

Marie glanced at the screen. There was only one cat.

"See them dancing?"

"I only see one cat, honey, and it's not moving."

"No, there are a lot of them," said Tina, turning toward Marie. Then she broke into laughter even louder than before. "How do you do that, Mommy? There are so many of you. It's funny, Mommy. How do you do it?"

My God, thought Marie. Something's wrong with her vision. She hurried to her daughter's side and began checking vital signs. Her pulse and respiration were slow. The child was having trouble keeping her eyes open and her speech was becoming slurred. If she didn't know better, she'd say her daughter was suffering from some sort of poisoning.

"Tina, are there still several of me?"

Tina's eyes were closing but she forced them open long enough to glance at her mother. "Yes, Mommy. It's fun ..." Her voice trailed off into an incomprehensible jumble of sounds. Her eyes closed tightly and her body went limp. Her breathing was shallow and, though Marie had no idea what was happening to the child, she was certain that if she didn't get help immediately, her daughter might die.

Marie grabbed Tina in her arms and ran to the car. She's eaten something, thought Marie, starting the engine and racing down the street toward the hospital emergency room. She's taken something bad for her. Maybe my pills. My God, she knows better than to take things from the medicine chest, but with a child, who can tell. Oh, my God ... My God ...

The trip to the hospital took just a few minutes. Marie kept pressing the accelerator to the floor, darting in and out of traffic, barely pausing at lights and stop signs. Her only thought was to reach the emergency room where Tina could get help.

The hospital's nursing staff rushed Tina into a room where the doctors could examine her. Ipecac was ordered to induce vomiting while Marie was questioned about what happened.

Marie was numb from shock. The doctor kept asking her about medication but all she could recall was the Methaqualone she kept in the medicine chest. She was certain Tina would never take that, but when the doctor checked a guide to medication, he discovered that Tina's reaction was typical of someone overdosing on that particular drug.

Why would she take those pills? thought Marie. She knows she's not supposed to touch them and she's always such a good child. She's never done anything like this before.

Maybe I should have watched her more closely. Maybe I've been spending too much time away from her. She might be doing all sorts of things I know nothing about.

There was no thought of personal involvement. Marie

could accept the idea that she might have deliberately injured herself but it was totally beyond her belief system to think she might have hurt Tina. Marie adored her daughter. She was the one person who brought her total joy. She knew it would have been impossible for her to have somehow given Tina access to the medication.

Looking back, I think this incident was the final straw. Charlene was no longer there to absorb this kind of shock for Marie, and she was more or less incapable of coping with the stress that Charlene had always borne. I had already resigned myself to the loss of Guido's children; Tina was the most important relationship in my life. The close call was enough to make Marie lose her already tenuous control over the body. And Linda was more than ready to take the reins. Ultimately, she would drive herself to destruction.

Linda waited until Leonard was asleep, then went to where he kept the checkbook and took some checks.

Linda got in her car as soon as Len left the house. She drove to the drive-in windows of four different branches of the bank where Len had his account. Each time she cashed a check for the maximum amount she thought she could get without the teller doing any checking of the account. She chose the drive-in windows so she could make a quick getaway if there was any trouble. Everything went smoothly, however. The signatures she forged were accepted without question. She drove away from the last bank, a total of $400 richer than when she had started her visits an hour earlier.

The checking account was wiped clean as the result of the four checks, but Linda had several blanks remaining. Len had good credit at two nearby bars so Linda stopped at one, getting another $100.

High on pills, she headed downtown, visiting clothing and department stores. She bought everything that struck her fancy, paying with the stolen checks. Although the account had been emptied, she managed to get her checks accepted without anyone investigating to see if she had sufficient funds, since Marie had always been known for having good credit. For three days she shopped, popped pills, and passed bad checks.

It was the third day of Linda's adventure and she decided she would leave for San Diego where there would be more "action." She still had plenty of money from the forged checks. She knew Len could make good on the account and she firmly believed he would. At 7 P.M. there was a knock on her motel room door.

Linda jerked open the door and was surprised to see two sheriff's deputies who worked at the jail with Marie. She smiled when she recognized them and invited them inside.

"Marie, I don't know how to tell you this," said one of the deputies. "We have orders to take you to the station with us." He didn't say he was arresting her, nor did he read Linda her rights.

When Linda went on her spending spree, Len called a friend of his from school days. The friend, who directed an alcoholic detoxification center, had seen Linda at her best and at her worst. Both men assumed that alcoholism and drug abuse were her only problems, never dreaming they were dealing with a multiple personality. They talked about the situation and consulted a third man who worked for Children's Protective Services. Together they decided that since Linda/Marie would never voluntarily seek help, it was time for her to be forced into a situation where help could be ordered for her. As a result, Len filed a complaint with the police, knowing that the judge could be persuaded to insist upon rehabilitative care rather than jail. He figured that if she could stay dry a few weeks, her problems would be over.

Linda smiled as he talked. She could tell the deputies were uncomfortable about picking her up. They had always been quite friendly with Marie when she worked at the jail and appreciated what she tried to do for the prisoners.

It was going to be a game, Linda realized as she got into the patrol car. She was going to manipulate the pigs the way she manipulated everybody. She'd have them kissing her ass before the evening was over and then she'd split the city.

The matron was surprised to see Linda and didn't bother taking her to the main booking area, even though she knew Linda was being charged with a crime. Instead she took her to the matron's quarters down a hallway to the right. She and all the other staff members wanted to treat her as a friend.

The booking procedure went quickly. Four sets of fingerprints were taken for filing with the FBI, the state capital, the local sheriff's office, and an arrest jacket, as her local record was called. This was followed by photos of her, full face and right profile.

Then she called a bondsman and bailed herself out.

The next morning Linda packed her bags, checked her resources, and left for San Diego. First she went to three different jewelry stores shortly after they opened and bought rings which cost a total of $2,500. She used some of the remaining blank checks on which she had forged her husband's signature. The rings could be hocked if she needed cash quickly and enjoyed on her fingers if she could remain solvent otherwise.

Linda planned to stay with her sister, Miriam, and Miriam's husband who lived in San Diego. Their contact over the years had been minimal. There were the usual Christmas cards and birthday remembrances. An occasional phone call or letter had also passed between them (between Marie and Miriam, anyway). But despite the infrequency of their communication, Linda knew her sister would have a place for her. Miriam had a strong sense of family. The three children had been at each other's throats more often than not, but their experience with their father had given them an unusual bond.

Linda called Miriam as soon as she reached San Diego. The visit was totally unexpected, yet the only question Miriam asked was whether her sister was alone or with Len and/or Tina. Linda explained that she was alone and Miriam told her to come right out to the house.

Linda checked her purse before going to Miriam's home. She was addicted to phenobarbital by then and knew she would be needing more in the next few days to avoid the pain of withdrawal. She hoped she had an adequate supply with her, but, as she feared, it was almost all gone. She had to convince Miriam to not only let her stay with her but also to help her get more of the drug.

"I have a bad heart," Linda told Miriam. "Do you think you could help me get an appointment with your family doctor so I can get another prescription for down here? If I don't do it soon, I'm going to be in real trouble."

The last statement wasn't a lie. Linda would be in trouble without her medication but it wasn't her heart that would be affected. An addict who suddenly stopped taking phenobarbital suffered withdrawal effects that were every bit as painful as those experienced by heroin addicts.

The next morning, the two of them went to Miriam's doctor. Linda lied, telling the doctor she didn't need an examination as she had had one before leaving Santa Cruz. That was where the heart problem was diagnosed, she explained, and the doctor believed her. He gave her a new prescription.

Linda was preoccupied with escaping reality. She wanted to be "high" no matter what she was doing.

Miriam had a swimming pool and Linda thought it would be fun to go floating in the water. But even this relaxing activity had to be heightened by taking a large dose of Nembutal before climbing into the pool. She never considered the effect the drug might have on someone in the water and that proved an almost fatal mistake.

Suddenly the sky and the water seemed to be one. As Linda stared, fascinated, the sky fell down upon her. It wrapped her body in its blueness and cut off her air. But Linda didn't panic. The drug had dulled her senses to the point where she failed to realize that, in reality, she had slipped below the surface of the chlorinated water. She continued to breathe normally, her lungs emptying of air and filling with water as she smiled happily.

Fortunately Miriam had seen her sister sink below the surface of the water. With the help of her twelve-year-old son, Miriam managed to drag Linda from the pool and give her artificial respiration.

Miriam checked on Linda throughout the night and, when she finally awakened, Miriam brought her a tray of food. Linda ate everything, then took several more Nembutal capsules to help get her through the morning. She lit a cigarette and leaned back against the pillow to enjoy it.

I have no idea what happened next. Linda's drug-fogged brain was so confused that my memory of the incident remains incomplete even now that my personalities have fused. All I know for certain is that suddenly the bed was on fire and I was facing a wall of flames. One of my alter-personalities began screaming and the next thing I remember is the room filling with people and water. Someone lifted me off my feet and carried me to safety.

Oh, my God. Where am I? Where the hell am I? thought Marie, looking frantically about the living room in which she was seated. The furnishings were familiar, yet they weren't her own.

"There you are, Marie," said Miriam, coming up behind her sister. Marie whirled to face her, an expression of shocked horror on her face.

"I just wanted to make certain you were all right," said Miriam. "You gave us quite a scare with that fire in your bedroom. Just getting some fresh air?"

Marie stared at her sister. Had Miriam come to see her or

was she really in San Diego? Maybe that was why the furnishings were familiar. She was in Miriam's home, a place she had visited upon occasion over the past few years. But why had she gone there? And how had she traveled? Was Len there? Or Tina? Or... My God, this is the worst the blackouts have ever been. Miriam was hundreds of miles away from where she lived, yet...

"What's the matter, Marie? Is it your heart again? Do you need your medicine? You don't look well at all."

Medicine? My heart? What's she talking about? "I'm all right. It's just..."

Marie attempted to calm herself. If she could regain an outward appearance of being relaxed, she could work the conversation around to where she might be able to learn what was happening.

It's getting worse. I'm getting longer blackout spells and the things I'm doing are more radical. My God, does this mean that one day I'll start living my whole life without any knowledge of it? Will I start going for weeks or months or even years without a conscious awareness?

Maybe this will work out for the best, thought Marie. Maybe I do need a major change in my life and San Diego's as good a place to start as any. I can find a job, then get settled and bring Tina to live with me. After that, Len and I can work out our problems.

The next morning Marie began job hunting in earnest, her sister driving her from hospital to hospital and medical office to medical office. Job opportunities for nurses were plentiful in the San Diego area that year and, by the end of the day, Marie was employed as a nurse for the Red Cross. The job was at a donor station where she would draw blood. Marie thought she might enjoy the work, at least for the moment, but she never realized she wouldn't spend even one day on the job.

Marie was elated as Miriam drove her home from the Red

Cross. They parked in the garage, then walked into the house. To their surprise, Miriam's husband was sitting and talking with two men dressed in conservative gray suits, white shirts, and brightly colored ties.

"Are you Marie Peters?" asked one of the men. They had stood up when she entered the room.

"Yes," said Marie, a puzzled smile on her face.

The man took a card from his pocket and began reading. "You are being placed under arrest. You have the right to remain silent. You have the right to an attorney. If you cannot afford an attorney, one will be appointed for you. If you decide to say anything, it can and . . ."

Marie was placed in the back seat of the detectives' car. It had been parked several houses from where Miriam lived so it would not be observed. There was no partition between the front and back seat so Marie was able to reach her cuffed hands over the side. She painfully maneuvered her hands so she could work the rings from her fingers. Then she gave the rings to the detective sitting on the passenger side, saying, "I suppose you'll be wanting these." He accepted the rings without comment.

Tears streamed down Marie's face. All her life she had managed to avoid serious trouble, even though she knew something was wrong with her mind. But in the past, everyone had accepted what she had done.

Now all that was changing. Once again she had done something she didn't remember and this time it was more serious. This time no one was going to laugh it off.

Man, did these two pigs scare the living shit out of that asshole Marie, thought Linda, smiling to herself. She looked out the window of the detectives' car as it made its way through traffic. I don't know what she's so afraid of. So they arrested her. Hell, I got out of the other jail in no time flat and I can do it down here, too.

The car pulled into downtown San Diego and began passing bars, liquor stores, shops, and other businesses. In the distance was a building that obviously was a government structure. It was old, gray, and several stories high. It was the police station, and in a few minutes the booking process would be started. Linda knew it would be dull. She didn't want to waste time going through that damned routine. She decided to let Marie take over again.

Marie was frightened as she was led through a series of ground-level offices, then into a room where two matrons were standing. The officers removed the handcuffs and left the room.

"Take off your clothes," said the larger of the two matrons. Actually she was several inches shorter than the other woman, but she compensated for her lack of height by having an excess of bulk. She had mountainous breasts which flopped against a stomach large enough to be used as an advertising billboard. Her stringy black hair looked as though it had been purchased from a used-wig shop. She looked like she could break someone's back with a twist of her fat fingers, and Marie knew better than to try and argue with her about anything.

"Yes, of course," said Marie. "Where do you want me to strip?" She blushed from embarrassment but was ready to cooperate fully.

The matron pointed to a small room shielded from view by a curtain hanging from an aged rod. Marie left her coat and purse on a table, then went into the smaller room to undress. She took off everything but her undergarments.

"Take off the bra and panties, too," said the matron. Then she gathered all Marie's belongings, put them into a bag, and took them from the room. Marie remained stark naked, terrified by what was happening. It was one thing to take care of prisoners in the jail, quite another to be one of them.

The matron returned to where Marie was standing. She slipped on a thin surgical glove and said, "Okay, bend over."

Marie bent at the waist. "Not that way," said the matron. "Squat!"

Suddenly Marie felt the matron's hand exploring her anus and her vagina. The matron was searching her private parts for hidden drugs. It was horrible—humiliating. Marie seemed to be able to feel the hand even after it was withdrawn. She had heard inmates in the jail complain about this type of search but she never experienced one before, even as a witness. The sensation of it seemed worse than the idea of being in jail. She wondered why anyone who had experienced it would ever commit a crime again.

"Grunt like you're having a bowel movement," said the matron.

Marie was shocked. "I've got nothing inside of me," she said. "I have no intention of grunting and if you can't tell that I'm not carrying anything without my making a stupid noise, that's your problem."

The matron finished her search, angered by the lack of cooperation. She gave Marie the prison uniform—a cotton sack dress, cotton underpants, and no bra. Marie was also issued rubber thongs.

Marie was neither fingerprinted nor photographed because a teletype from Santa Cruz alerted the jail officials that this had already been done. She was told she could make one telephone call and could take one unopened pack of cigarettes with her into the next room. All other personal property was stored away.

During this period, Marie gradually learned why she was being held in jail. She realized that she was a bail jumper but didn't know the seriousness of that crime. She doubted that she was in much trouble since she heard that her previous bail had been $1,000. Obviously her thefts, if that's what they were, had been minor. Certainly she hadn't killed anyone.

A higher bail was set once Marie illegally left Santa Cruz. The same judge who had released her for $1,000 set the new bail, under which San Diego authorities were holding her, at $50,000. To make matters worse, Miriam, the only person who could help her in San Diego, refused to put up the $5,000 necessary to insure her release. Miriam realized that there was more to her sister than she had known; $5,000 was a small fortune to Miriam and she couldn't risk gambling it on a sister she discovered she didn't really understand. Marie was trapped in prison.

This is the beginning of the end, thought Marie. All my life I've been faking and getting away with it. Now I know why crazy people always end their lives in institutions. They do something bad which they can't explain, like whatever crimes I must have committed in Santa Cruz.

How can I hope to defend myself? I can plead guilty and go to jail or I can explain to the judge that I have no idea what I do or where I go much of the time. He won't send me to jail if he believes that. He'll just lock me away in an asylum.

To make the waiting even more frightening, the jail holding area in which Marie found herself contained the strangest assortment of women she had ever seen. There were prostitutes for whom jail was like a second home. There were drug addicts lying on the floor, curled into a ball, sweating and screaming, while other addicts, not yet experiencing the pain of withdrawal, watched in terror of what they, too, would soon endure. There were bank robbers, murderers, and women who had committed every crime imaginable.

The noise, the smells, and the tension of the holding cell overwhelmed Marie. She was fearful of the other inmates, for whom, in many cases, violence was a natural part of life. She huddled in a corner of the cell, her head spinning and her eyes closed. A moment later she was gone.

Holy shit! When you've seen one of these rat traps, you've seen them all, thought Linda.

Linda patted her clothes, looking for a cigarette. What is this? No smokes and a $50,000 bail.

Well, if I can't get out of this joint, the least I can do is raise a little hell around here, thought Linda. Yet looking back from the perspective of a mentally whole individual, I can't help but wonder if there wasn't more to Linda's reasoning. It seems as though my subconscious mind was desperately crying out for help. I couldn't continue in the nightmare existence my alters were leading, yet neither Linda nor Marie were ready to seek help directly.

Linda went over to the toilet and noticed a thin wire in a mechanism. It was just what she needed.

It took several minutes to free the wire but no one seemed to have noticed or cared about what Linda was doing. When she finally had it, she took one end and began slashing at her throat. She ripped the flesh, pushing the tip of the wire into her skin, then tearing across. The wire was sharp enough to cut her throat and cause extensive bleeding.

The women in the cell saw the bleeding and shouted for the guards who quickly took the wire from Linda's hand. She began lashing out at the men who were trying to subdue her, but they were too quick for her. They managed to get her restrained and on a stretcher with a minimum of fuss.

Linda was kept in the hospital for the next few days, her wrists and legs constantly in restraints. She was considered too dangerous both to herself and the staff to let her go free. When her wounds were healing well, she was returned to jail.

Enough of this shit, thought Linda.

Marie came slowly to consciousness. She was still on heavy medication, both to keep her calm and to fight infection from her wounds. The drugs hadn't fazed Linda. Alcohol and narcotics were no match for the body chemistry Linda seemed to generate. But when Marie was in control, everything changed. Drugs affected her as they were supposed to, and the medicine the hospital doctors had prescribed kept her quite groggy at first.

Everything's different, Marie realized as she sat up on the hard, thin mattress that served as her bed. The people have changed. I'm not with the same women I was when I lay down.

Marie wanted to talk with the other prisoners to find out if her suspicions were correct. But before she could question anyone, one of the guards noticed she was awake and moved her to a single cell. The barbiturates she was carrying, the same ones she had originally obtained in San Diego, had been discovered. It was assumed, correctly, that she would soon go through the agony of withdrawal. It would be easiest on the other prisoners if she did it in a cell by herself.

As soon as the symptoms of withdrawal began, Marie was left completely alone. No one came to change the dressings on her wound. No one offered to bring her food. She had nothing to drink but the water from a sink in a corner of the cell.

For two days Marie experienced the agony of stopping barbiturates "cold turkey." She had pain, cramps, and nausea. Her face was flushed with a high fever. Sometimes she screamed and thrashed about the cell. Other times she lay curled in a fetal position, moaning and hugging her body. Still other times she fell into a troubled sleep, only to be awakened by uncontrollable convulsions and sweat pouring down her face. The guards were neither sympathetic nor concerned.

When a guard finally did check on Marie, it was not to learn about her condition but rather to see if she was willing to be flown back to Santa Cruz. She could be driven or flown and, while flying was faster and more convenient for the jail staff, many prisoners didn't like it. The courts had ruled that prisoners could refuse to be flown without such a refusal hurting their cases or resulting in punishment.

Marie insisted upon being driven back to her home county. She was not trying to cause any trouble but suffered from a fear of heights so severe that she couldn't even look over the side of a low bridge without becoming nauseated.

The guard who questioned Marie about the trip left her cell without bothering to check her injuries. Had she done so, she would have seen that the wound had become badly infected. It was draining a foul-smelling thick yellow pus. Most of the dressings had worn away and the only relief Marie got came from wrapping the injury with the thin, slime-covered gray blanket that was issued for bedding.

Several days after Marie's arrest in San Diego, a matron and a Sheriff's Department deputy arrived from Santa Cruz to take her back to their county jail. All three were acquainted with one another but the spirit of friendship following that first arrest was no longer in evidence. Suddenly Marie had become "big time" because of her escape and the resultant increase in bail. They showed her neither favoritism nor friendliness. No matter what they thought of her before, now she had become as bad as any other criminal in their eyes.

Marie dressed in the clothing she was wearing when arrested—a white nurse's uniform, white shoes and hose as well as her nursing school pin. Only her purse and personal jewelry were retained by the deputy.

Marie thought she would ride back to Santa Cruz as a passenger in the patrol car sent to pick her up. She was mistaken. To her horror, the deputy and the matron placed her in special leg shackles which forced her to take short, mincing steps. Her wrists were handcuffed together. Then a wide, heavy leather belt was strapped around her waist and additional handcuffs were used to link each wrist to the belt. The only way she could scratch her nose was by doubling her body. They were the same precautions used when transporting a mass murderer.

Walking from the jail, through the open parking lot to the Sheriff's Department car was the most humiliating experience Marie had ever known. Even worse, she would not be free from her bonds for the next ten hours—the time for the drive back to Santa Cruz.

Halfway through the trip, the sheriff's deputy pulled the car into the parking lot of a Denny's Restaurant. He and the matron were hungry and they knew the county would pay for their meals. "Come on," said the matron. "Let's go eat."

Marie wasn't particularly hungry but she was delighted by the prospect of being freed from her chains for a while. She held out her hands, expecting the matron to unlock the cuffs.

The matron opened the car door and gestured for Marie to get out. She made no effort to unlock the cuffs. Apparently Marie was expected to walk shackled into the restaurant, a freak at whom all the customers would stare.

"You've got to be putting me on!" said Marie, shocked and hurt by the treatment. They also seemed to want to humiliate her. They were like the owners of a dog whose nose was being constantly pushed into piles of his shit.

In fairness to the deputy and the matron, Linda's violent actions would normally have warranted such careful restraint in order to protect them. But Marie was totally incapable of doing anything criminal or violent. Keeping her shackled while in uniform was cruel punishment; worse than any prison sentence a judge could hand out.

"You really expect me to go in there like this?" asked Marie, beginning to cry again.

"Sure, why not?" said the deputy. He thought of the warning he had been given by his superiors before he left for San Diego. Marie was capable of changing from a gentle person to a violent one in a matter of seconds. No matter what she had been like when working as the jail nurse, she was no longer to be trusted.

Marie said nothing. How could they not understand her feelings? She glared at the deputy and matron and refused to move. Reluctantly they returned to the car and drove to a carry-out hot dog stand. To Marie's delight, they got indigestion from the spicy meat. She chose to have black coffee only and her stomach felt fine when they reached the jail.

The staff of the Santa Cruz county jail seemed embarrassed when Marie hobbled into the holding area. No matter how much respect they had lost for her when she jumped bail, they were ashamed at the way she was forced to appear before them.

The jail admission procedure was more familiar to Marie after her experience in San Diego. Stoop down . . . Check the vagina . . . Check the anus . . . Leave your clothes . . . Leave your possessions . . . Put on regulation jeans and sweatshirt . . . Go here . . . Go there . . . Into the cage with the rest of the animals.

After booking was completed, one of the matrons, a close friend from Marie's nursing days, happened to spot her. She took Marie into the matron's office and there were tears in her eyes. She told Marie how sorry she was for the treatment Marie was getting. "Whatever you've done, honey, it couldn't have warranted your being chained like that."

The matron gave Marie a cigarette. Marie took it gratefully, lighting it, then slowly inhaling and exhaling the smoke in order to calm her nerves.

"Take your time with the cigarette," said the matron. "I won't put you in the cell until you've had a chance to calm down. Can I get you a cup of coffee?"

"I'd love one," said Marie. She suddenly realized she was tired. She had slept during most of the drive to the jail but it had not been restful. She was also suffering from the emotional strain of the experience and felt so humiliated she didn't want to continue. She shut her eyes for a moment. When they opened, they were alive with fire.

The matron's office, thought Linda, looking around the room. I ought to be able to spring us out of here.

Linda noticed the desk where bags containing her belongings were placed. Among them was an envelope with all the drugs found in Marie's purse. Linda glanced down the hall to see if the matron was coming back, then ripped open the envelope, took out the phenobarbital and swallowed as many as she could.

Nobody's going to lock me up like a monkey in a zoo, thought Linda as she waited for the drug to work. Hospitals were better than jails. You had more freedom and, if you played your cards right, you could just walk out.

I won't take all the pills. I'll save a small handful for the matron to see. The poor slob will think she caught me before I could take any and go around saying she saved my life.

The matron returned with the coffee, found the pills, and gave Linda a lecture. No matter how bad things seemed, the matron said, there was always hope. Taking pills to try and kill herself was the wrong way to cope.

Linda sipped the coffee and nodded her agreement, letting the matron think she had returned in time to stop a suicide attempt. When Linda finished her coffee, she was taken to a cell where she lay down on the floor. She knew she would awaken either in the hospital or wherever she was going to go after this life, depending on whether or not she was discovered in time. It didn't matter which.

Marie awakened in a hospital room. Her head ached and she had trouble seeing. All she could tell was that she was no longer in the matron's office or any other part of the jail. She did not know that she had been in a coma for fourteen hours in the jail cell and that her body had turned blue before the other inmates were able to convince the jailer she needed emergency treatment. Once again she had barely escaped dying and had no idea what had happened.

Barbiturate withdrawal was especially hard on Marie, who was not able to tolerate much pain. Charlene did not come out. I don't know if she wanted to punish Marie for not getting help or if she felt that the adult Marie should tolerate pain from which the younger Marie would have been protected. When Marie could no longer stand the cramps, the nausea, and the other problems, it was Linda who took control of the body.

Linda was shocked by the pain. She was angry that Marie was so weak as to be unable to stay in control of the body during its period of agony. Marie had to be punished.

The guards had taken out all possibly dangerous implements, but they left a ball point pen. Linda quickly took out the gold-colored metal refill, broke it in half with her teeth, then made a jagged edge by repeatedly biting the soft metal.

I'll give those mothers something to remember, thought Linda. She covered herself with her blanket, then began sawing at her arm. She exposed the vein, artery, and nerve, working so slowly that the average person would have collapsed from the pain. Linda felt nothing, however. She had a single purpose in mind, and a little pain wasn't going to stop her from reaching it.

Before Linda could slice through the artery, the matron spotted her huddled figure and realized Linda was doing something under the blanket that she didn't want anyone to see.

"What have you got there?" asked the matron.

"Nothing," said Linda.

The matron didn't believe her. She looked closer, spotting

the blood that had been running down Linda's arm. Shocked by the sight, the matron rushed down the hall to get the jailers. She knew Linda needed emergency care.

Linda realized that even if she slashed open her artery, she could not bleed to death before people came to restrain her. She looked frantically about, then spotted a bottle of lanolin shampoo. She rushed to it, unscrewed the cap, and drank it down. The taste must have been extremely unpleasant but Linda was unaware of its "flavor."

The jailers rushed Linda to the hospital once again. Her arm was stitched back together and she was treated for the internal damage from the shampoo. Then she was taken to a room where she fell asleep, her body exhausted from the trauma.

When Linda returned to the jail, she decided to let Marie have control of the body. This was fortunate because the court had ordered two psychiatric evaluations of her. One of the psychiatrists was Dr. Brewster.

The session with Dr. Brewster took place on March 9, 1973. This time Marie, not Linda, was the personality meeting him. Dr. Brewster still appeared disheveled, but he seemed friendlier and more human to Marie than he had to Linda.

That meeting was not very dramatic. Marie answered the questions that were on a form used by Dr. Brewster for this type of court-required interview. She spoke honestly about her drinking and drug habits. However, she did not feel comfortable enough to volunteer information. Dr. Brewster asked nothing about her memory losses, so she kept quiet about them. She could not bring herself to ask for his help.

Dr. Brewster looked upon the interview as being no different from hundreds of others he had conducted over the years. To him, Marie was another alcoholic. He found her sensitive and able to cry readily when her feelings were hurt. He reported her statement that her ability to think and reason was about 55 percent of normal and improving daily after the last hospitalization.

Dr. Brewster concluded that Marie's problems were limited to alcoholism and barbiturate addiction. He felt she was capable of standing trial and could best be helped in a residential treatment facility. The idea of multiple personality never entered his mind.

10

COMING TOGETHER

The next few months were to prove a nightmare world of self-destructive acts. It was as though Linda sensed that perhaps help was possible and that her future existence was in jeopardy. Whether it was something in Dr. Brewster's manner during that brief interview session for the court or some other experience, something seemed to threaten Linda. She knew that if she didn't attack the body, Marie would somehow triumph, and she couldn't have that.

Marie also seemed to sense a change coming in her life. She lost interest in her work and began drinking heavily herself. She seemed to abandon hope of a normal life, yet tried to hang on for something in the future which she sensed more than actually understood. However, she and Linda had to touch bottom, after many months of dope, sex, and booze, before she would finally grab hold of the "life raft" known as Dr. Brewster.

Linda and Marie, sharing the body, stayed in the Santa Cruz jail four months, during which time several court appearances were made. None of the judges seemed to be certain just what to do with me at first. Finally it was decided that the problem was drug addiction and that release to a halfway house for drug addicts was the most sensible way to deal with me.

It was ironic that the judge focused on the drug abuse. Both Linda and Marie were alcoholics and had been for a considerable length of time. The addiction to pills had been going on just a few months and wasn't nearly so serious.

The recommended treatment seemed designed to put a greater strain on my alter-personalities than they had endured before. Marie was to stay in the halfway house for three months without seeing husband or child. She was dependent on both of them for support. There was no one else she could depend on or relate to. Her life was becoming meaningless. The nursing jobs were almost nonexistent and there was nothing else to keep her functioning except the knowledge that she had to meet the needs of her daughter and husband.

I'm all alone out here, thought Marie, looking around the rural home where she would be the only female patient housed with five male patients. Nobody needs me. Nobody really wants me. It doesn't matter whether I live or die. Everything will go on as it always has.

Why do they keep harassing me? thought Marie as she began experiencing the halfway house "treatment" which was expected to cure her. The staff believed that her ego should be totally destroyed. She was expected to develop the attitude that everything she did was meaningless so she could be remolded as they saw fit.

The longer Marie stayed in the halfway house, the more she came to realize that the "professionals" didn't have the slightest idea what they were doing.

Once, for example, approximately six weeks after Marie began living at the halfway house, she was driven into the city for a "therapy session" in a second house which served as offices for the group. Two dirty mattresses and a large, shaggy rug comprised the total furnishings in the room to which she was taken. The walls were peeling, stained, and smelled of mold.

Three women and a man joined her.

A female counselor entered the room and everyone acted as though programmed. As Marie watched, they took off their clothing, leaving on only their undergarments.

Everyone ignored Marie. They positioned themselves on the mattresses and the floor, then began rocking their bodies, emitting low moans. They moved about, quivering and shaking.

The counselor, her face flushed with excitement, explained to Marie that it was a treatment concept known as bioenergetic therapy.

The counselor seemed to sense Marie's uneasiness. "Don't let it worry you. You'll get used to it. I'm going to sign you up for one class a week and you'll soon be just as much a part of it as the others."

"No way," said Marie. "It's nothing personal, you understand, but there's no way I'm going to participate in a group like that."

Later Marie learned that the staff had amended her chart to indicate that she was not being cooperative. Still, that was better than acting like a crazy person one day each week.

Ultimately, because she was considered uncooperative, the staff attempted to get rid of her. She was listed as a disruptive influence who would not benefit from the halfway house environment. As a result, the court ordered her to return home under a strict set of rules laid down by the probation department.

In early 1974, Marie got the last meaningful job she was able to hold. She was hired by a doctor who was a specialist in metabolic nutrition. He had all the credentials of a "proper" medical doctor but was considered a maverick in the medical community. He felt that correct diet could do more to prevent and/or relieve illness than all the medications available. Many of his patients came to him after normal medical treatment failed and their doctors told them there was no hope. However, by changing their diet and using vitamins rather than pills, he restored most to a state of health they had been told was impossible to achieve again.

The patients came from all over the United States, as

the doctor was widely known through his books and magazine articles. He hired Marie to learn his methods so that she could work closely with the patients, supplying them with advice and information after they had been given extensive tests and started on an individualized program by the doctor.

The doctor was also a deeply religious man who had a Bible study session in his office every morning before work. He applied his religious beliefs to his employee relationships and was always ready to welcome Marie after Linda took off for several days of drinking without notifying the doctor she wouldn't be in.

Before going to work for the doctor, Marie was assigned to a probation officer named Sara Carlson. Sara was hostile toward anyone she considered weak. She had only disdain for people who drank too much or constantly took pills. Since Marie's case indicated her felonies resulting from drug addiction, she decided to make Marie pay in every way possible.

Sara announced that if Marie wanted to return to nursing, she had to first tell an employer her entire background. Next she would have to undergo urinalysis several times a week to be certain there were no traces of barbiturates in her body. Then she was to tell any doctor for whom she worked that she was not to be placed in a position where she would be handling medicine. In other words, Marie could wear a nurse's uniform and make sympathetic noises to the patients but she couldn't perform the duties for which she had been trained.

I can't take it anymore, thought Marie at the end of May, 1974. I'm the kind of person who needs to feel in control of her life. I need to get away, to escape, to be free...

Marie did escape, letting Linda take control of the body while she retreated into the mind. But Linda was fast reaching bottom herself.

I hate this shit, thought Linda. I've got to get everybody off my back.

Linda called the doctor for whom Marie had been working and quit her job, giving neither reasons nor notice. She, too, wanted to escape, but for her the bottle was the answer. She no longer wanted good times, excitement, and men. She was miserable and didn't know why. The only thing that eased the depression was the booze, and she scrounged everywhere to get enough money for yet another bottle. She stole pennies, nickels, and dimes from her daughter's piggy bank and from anywhere Len was foolish enough to leave a little money.

One night the liquor ran out but not the desire for escape. Linda, barefoot and wearing a thin housecoat, left the house under cover of darkness while Len slept unaware. She made her way along the road, passing horses grazing in pastures and businesses locked and darkened for the night. Eventually she reached a liquor store several miles from the house. The six-foot-square display window was made of heavy glass, but a brick Linda hurled against it proved it wasn't unbreakable. She reached inside, grabbed two fifths of brandy from the shelves by reaching through the broken glass, then ran. She stopped to take an occasional swallow but didn't get serious about her drinking until she was safe at home. Although she had heard police sirens, she had not been spotted by the investigating patrolman who responded to the store's burglar alarm.

The days and weeks blurred together. Marie was drinking almost as heavily as Linda because she didn't know what else to do. It was the first time she considered that admitting her problem might be better than the life she was leading. Being locked away in a mental ward might not be any more restrictive than being controlled by Sara and the bottle. And there was that slim chance that there were answers; that someone might be able to help her.

Then Marie discovered to what depths she had sunk. She was found with her head lying in a vase partially filled with the vomit she was trying to save for its alcoholic content. When she regained consciousness, she was ready to get help.

I never did learn what Dr. Brewster thought of me that first day in the hospital. He remembered Marie from his earlier contacts but always seemed unwilling to help her because she refused to make any effort toward changing the existence she was leading. Like many psychiatrists, he had been victimized by patients in the past who claimed to want his help but were really playing games with themselves. Alcoholics, for example, might arrange for psychiatric therapy to help them overcome their addiction, then say the stress of the appointments forced them to drink all the more. He assumed Marie was that type, as her name had appeared on hospital admissions records so frequently.

The doctor couldn't stay with Marie after helping her back into her room the day she finally asked for help, but he promised to return after he was finished with his regular patients. By the time he came back, an hour of two later, Linda was in charge.

Asshole's gone and done it again. Now I've got to put up with that rooster, Brewster.

When Dr. Brewster returned, Linda began telling him of all her troubles. She said she was in pain and unable to sleep. "I've got to get some rest or I'll die; I swear I'll die." She was watching his face to see if anything she said or did had an effect on him, but he never changed. He remained impassive.

"I don't think pills are the answer," said Dr. Brewster. "They have their place in treatment, but your record shows you've had a few too many. Have you ever thought of hypnosis?"

"Of what?"

"Hypnosis. It's a legitimate tool used by many psychiatrists. I used it to help focus the mind and narrow concentration to a limited area. There's nothing magical about it and the so-called trance is really nothing more than a state of heightened, concentrated awareness. It can help you relax. I'd like to see if I can hypnotize you right now to give you rest."

"So what happens when I'm hypnotized, doc?" asked Linda. "What do you do with me then?"

"Nothing very mysterious. I'm going to make some suggestions that will help ease the pain so you can relax and get a good night's sleep without drugs. It's much safer for someone in your present condition."

I don't know about this, thought Linda. I don't like the idea of a man having that kind of control over me. I don't want someone else calling the shots while I'm helpless.

"Are you willing to try?" the doctor persisted.

"If I go ahead with it and it doesn't work, will you give me some medicine?"

"We'll see."

"All right. But this better be just the way you claim."

Dr. Brewster helped Linda to a chair. He ran some preliminary tests, such as an eye-roll test, to see if she was likely to be a good subject for hypnosis. When he had satisfied himself that she was, he said: "Close your eyes, Mrs. Peters. I want you to concentrate only on the darkness. Blot out all the distractions of the outside world. Just focus all your attention on the quiet inside your head."

Dr. Brewster spoke in a monotone, his droning voice having a soothing effect. Linda stopped gripping the arms of the chair and began to relax.

"I'm going to count to ten. When I'm through counting, you are going to be more relaxed than you have ever been before. Your pain will be gone and you are going to feel an inner peace."

And so Dr. Brewster put Linda under hypnosis. He worked quickly, not attempting to delve into her unconscious. He was trying only to relax her so he could use suggestions to eliminate her pain. When he brought her out, he commented, "Tonight you will sleep a peaceful sleep. Remember that and it will be so."

Linda had been skeptical of hypnosis but had cooperated enough to go into a light trance. She didn't want the doctor to have power over her, yet she couldn't see the harm in cooperating to some degree. As a result, the hypnotic suggestion worked and she slept better than she had in months.

The next day Marie awakened feeling better than she had felt for weeks. She wondered what sort of sleeping medication the nurses had given her but couldn't remember their doing it. Whatever it was, she felt truly rested.

Marie took a psychological test Dr. Brewster had ordered for her. She scored quite normally, a fact which further delayed Dr. Brewster's discovery that there was more wrong with this unusual woman than just alcoholism and drug abuse.

Len stopped by the hospital during visiting hours to bring Marie some cigarettes. The gesture surprised her as she didn't know her husband was aware she needed them. Actually, Linda had called him and raised hell because she had run out, insisting he bring her several packs.

After Len left the hospital, Linda took control and decided to create a little havoc. She called her home after waiting long enough for Len to have gotten back there. She learned that he had gone out for the evening.

"That no-good son of a bitch!" said Linda, slamming down the receiver. "I'm stuck in this place and that bastard is out carousing. Who the hell does he think he is to play around when I'm in the hospital?"

Linda began telephoning some of Len's friends, hoping to find one who knew where he might be. On the third call she learned that he and two other men were making the rounds of restaurants and bars they normally attended.

Linda called the first restaurant where she thought they would stop. Len had been there but left, though he was expected to return. "I have an important message for Mr. Peters," said Linda. "This is a nurse at the hospital. When Len comes back, please tell him to contact the hospital immediately at this number. His wife committed suicide. We need him to come right away and claim the body."

"Mrs. Peters died?" said the waitress who knew Len and Marie. "Oh, my God, are you sure? She was so young. This is terrible... Terrible... But don't worry. I'll tell Mr. Peters as soon as he comes back. I'll have him call you at once."

Linda had difficulty restraining her laughter until she had hung up the phone. The stupid-ass waitress had believed the line of shit she was handing out. She didn't know if Len would be that gullible, but she certainly hoped he would get a little upset at least. As it turned out, Len never got the message that had been left for him.

Linda didn't feel like staying in bed. She left her room and began walking the halls. Alcoholics drying out are left to themselves much of the time.

There was a storage closet down a hall and a utility room where supplies were kept. No one was around so Linda slipped inside, took a syringe and large needle from a tray, and hid them under her bathrobe.

Linda returned to her room, hid under the bed, and began slashing at her arm with the needle. She inserted it into one vein, then began drawing out the blood, in an attempt to empty her body of all its fluid.

The first shock was the pain. Marie grasped her arm, feeling as though someone had taken a hunting knife and plunged it through the flesh, muscles, and nerves. The pain was so intense she let out a piercing scream that seemed to echo off the walls and radiate through the halls.

Then Marie noticed the needle sticking into her arm and the thick blood caking on the skin around it. The syringe attached to the needle was filled with blood and the sheets were badly stained. She pulled the needle from her arm and hurled it against the far wall as a nurse rushed into the room to see why she had screamed. Together they cleaned and bandaged the wound, Marie unable to explain where she had gotten the syringe or why she had hurt herself with it.

The nurse wanted to either restrain Marie or give her a sedative to keep her from hurting herself further. There's a reason for this, thought Marie. Something's happening to me that I don't understand, but I know there's a reason. I can't just let myself get drugged into forgetting. I've got to know what's wrong.

"Dr. Brewster . . ." said Marie. "Please . . . call Dr. Brewster. He said to call him if I had any trouble. Don't do anything to me until I see if he can come here."

Marie was surprised when Dr. Brewster came to the hospital at once. It was late, well past the time when psychiatrists normally see their patients.

Dr. Brewster felt that when he became a psychiatrist, his primary duty was to his patients. If a patient was in trouble, he would leave his home in the middle of the night to take care of the person. He was a devoted family man, with a wife and four children, yet he always placed his patients above all other responsibilities. When Marie called him, sounding troubled and frightened, he decided that she might not be playing alcoholic games. She might genuinely be in need, and he felt compelled to go see her.

His concern really reached Marie. I've got to tell him everything. I can't be any worse off than I am. I don't want to get locked away for the rest of my life, yet if I'm not honest with him about my problems, I'm liable to be dead before I get any help. If he'll come to see me late at night like this, maybe he wouldn't put me away. I don't know. I just can't go on anymore. I've got to find out what's happening inside my head.

"Dr. Brewster, I feel terrible," said Marie, after the doctor arrived at her hospital room. "It's almost as though something's controlling me. Look at my arm. Can you imagine anyone doing all that to herself and not knowing it? I don't even remember getting hold of the needle and syringe. The first thing I knew, the needle was stuck in my arm and the pain was unbearable."

"There is one way to find out what happened," said Dr. Brewster. "I could put you in a trance and try to reach your memory that way. It would be the same as I did yesterday, only this time we would try and uncover what caused you to hurt yourself. It's a standard therapeutic technique and nothing to fear. It's just a way of getting into your mind when you are unable to consciously recall why you hurt yourself."

"All right, Dr. Brewster. Go ahead," said Marie, nervous about what the hypnosis would be like. Linda was the one who had been hypnotized earlier and Marie only had the doctor's word that he had done it before. Yet even though she was honest about some of her fears, she couldn't quite bring herself to admit she didn't remember the earlier hypnosis.

Dr. Brewster repeated the same basic instructions as before. Marie's body relaxed and she responded to each of his questions clearly and calmly.

"Marie, a few minutes before you called me, you took a syringe and needle and tried to draw out your blood. Why did you do that?"

"I didn't do that," said Marie.

"But you have wounds on your arm and you showed me the needle."

"I know. But I didn't do it. She did it."

Dr. Brewster later told me how startled he was by what Marie was saying. Normally the answers given under hypnosis are accurate.

"Who is this 'she' to whom you're referring? One of the nurses?"

"No. There's someone else. Someone in here with me."

Dr. Brewster had known of multiple personality ever since his medical school days and had treated a small number of patients with this problem. He had read all the literature available on the subject and retained an open mind concerning the condition. Yet because it is such an uncommon mental state, he refused to accept what was the obvious answer to my problem. He told me later that he wanted to explore all possibilities.

"Do you mean someone in this room?" said Dr. Brewster.

"No, I mean in here. In my head. There's someone else. She's the one who hurt me. She's the one who's always trying to hurt me."

"Does she have a name?"

"Yes. But I don't know what it is. I'm not around when she's doing things. I'm stuck inside and don't see what's happening."

"Well, can I talk with this other person?"

"I . . . I don't know. She's inside. She's . . ."

"Suppose you relax," said Dr. Brewster. "I'm going to take you deeper and I want you to relax."

Marie's body seemed almost to melt into the chair. Her face was serene and all tension completely vanished.

"Now I want to speak with the other one—the person who stabbed Marie's arm and tried to withdraw the blood. Come out and let me talk with you."

Suddenly Marie's eyes opened. They were harsh and glaring. Her lips changed to a half smile and she sat up on the chair, slipping her hospital gown up her thigh, crossing one leg over the other, and gently kicking the bare limb to call attention to it.

"What's the matter, doc? Get tired of that sniveling asshole? You wanted to talk to a real woman?"

"Are you the woman who used the syringe?"

"Hell, yes. What I really needed was a razor blade to cut the arm up good. But what the hell. You make do with what you've got, you know what I mean?"

"Why would you want to do that, Marie?"

"Shit, don't call me by *her* name!"

"Have we ever met?"

"Hell, we met a few years ago when I tried to kill myself, and I was the one you hypnotized that first time. I don't think I'd have let you do it if I'd of known you were going to mess around with me."

"What's your name?"

"Linda. And you'd damn well better remember it if you want to talk with me again."

"I'll definitely want to talk with you again, Linda. I'll want to talk with both you and Marie."

Linda laughed. "If you can find her," she said. "One of these days I'm going to send her straight to hell where she belongs."

"But if you hurt her, you're hurting yourself."

"Nothing bothers me, doc. I'll survive. She's the one who's going to suffer."

After a few more minutes, Dr. Brewster had Linda return to her section of the mind and brought Marie out of the trance. "Well, doctor, did I say anything interesting?" she asked hesitantly. She was still nervous about the hypnosis and concerned about what she might have said during the session.

"Yes . . . Yes, you did."

"What did I say? Did I tell you about the needle and syringe?"

"Yes, and I'm going to want to discuss this in some detail with you. I don't have time now, but I'm going to stop by tomorrow with some reading material for you that will explain things better than I can. Now don't worry about anything.

I've made some hypnotic suggestions to you again which will make it easy for you to sleep tonight. I'll be back as early as I can."

The following day Dr. Brewster presented the idea of multiple personality to Marie. He told her of the book *Sybil* and brought a number of articles that had been published about the phenomenon.

"I don't know for certain that this is your problem, Marie. There are a number of common factors in such cases and my talking with someone who called herself Linda does not, by itself, mean you are a multiple personality."

He explained some more about multiple personalities and what causes them.

"Dr. Brewster, I find this whole thing rather hard to believe," said Marie. "What you're talking about . . . I mean, I'd have to be a lunatic and I'm certain that's not the case."

"Multiple personality patients function well enough in the everyday world so that often their friends and family don't fully understand what's happening. They attribute the person's odd behavior to being 'moody' or 'eccentric' rather than a form of mental illness.

"Marie, does the name Linda mean anything to you?"

Marie's face paled and her hand trembled as she nervously picked at the arm of the chair. "Why . . . Why do you ask?"

"That was the name you gave me when you were under hypnosis. You said your name was Linda, not Marie, and that you, as Linda, were responsible for stabbing yourself with the syringe and needle."

People have called me Linda all my life, thought Marie. They joke about my liquor capacity and the obscene sex acts I supposedly performed when I know I never did any such things. Yet now Dr. Brewster's using that same name. But I can't be a multiple personality! I can't be! Such things don't happen to real people. I can't . . .

It would be several weeks before Marie could fully accept

the diagnosis of multiple personality. By then enough information had come out of the therapy sessions so that she could see how her life's pattern had followed the classic background of the "multiple." In the meantime, there were still many surprises in store for both Marie and Dr. Brewster.

As the hours passed that first day, Marie became increasingly uneasy. Victims of multiple personality are said to have hysterical dissociation. We are often highly imaginative individuals for whom fantasy and reality blend into one. When an alter-personality is first formed, it is often based on the imaginary playmate a child created when small. After the harsh triggering incident, the rape by my father in my case, the first personality is often the imaginary playmate made "real" in the child's mind.

Most children have imaginary playmates at some time in their lives and this is perfectly normal. It only becomes unhealthy when the playmate stops being "pretend" and takes on the characteristics of a real person. While I do not recall having such an imaginary playmate myself, I did have the same type of vivid imagination that is common to people with multiple personality.

For many years Marie had fantasized about spirits, the devil, witchcraft, and related matters. Some of this came from reading and seeing fantasy and science fiction stories. They provided a light escape from her troubles, just as did the nurse/romance stories she enjoyed.

The other reason Marie thought about witchcraft and spirits was because of the people she met in and out of the various mental wards. Many of these people had been searching for something outside themselves which they could use to get better. A number of them had practiced black magic and claimed to be devil worshippers. Others talked of spirits causing all their problems. Intellectually, Marie knew that such activities were ways the patients attempted to avoid accepting personal responsibility for their own actions. If they could convince others that something outside their body had forced them to do whatever acts resulted in their being institutionalized, then they might be freed. Emotionally, however, Marie wondered if such claims might not be true. She had seen people who mutilated and killed other human beings without a qualm, yet seemed gentle and sensitive at all other times. It was not hard to think of them as being "possessed" by something outside themselves when they committed their heinous crimes.

During this period, Marie was in Dominican Hospital rather than the county facility. Dominican was a church-affiliated institution open to the general public, and religious symbols were used among the decorations. Marie noticed a small wooden crucifix hanging on the wall. She grabbed the cross for whatever protection it might provide from "spirits and demons," then frantically called Dr. Brewster for help. It was late at night but she had to see him. Certainly she couldn't admit to any of the other staff people that she thought there were demons taking hold of her.

Dr. Brewster didn't ridicule her belief in possession. "It is a spirit of some kind, doctor," said Marie tearfully. "It's not that multiple personality thing at all. It's an evil spirit that is tormenting me. You've got to believe me. Dear God, I know it's true and you've got to believe me . . ."

"If you're convinced a spirit has possessed you, then it must be true," said Dr. Brewster. "Do you think that if you were rid of this spirit, you would be able to cooperate fully with me and start to get well?"

"Oh, yes, doctor. I know it. It's an evil spirit. I'm certain of that."

"Then all that's left for me to do now is exorcise that evil spirit."

"Can you do that?" asked Marie in astonishment.

"We psychiatrists have very special training. Besides, my

father is a minister and I once thought about entering the field myself. All God asks is that we believe in His curative powers, and if we do that, we can exorcise the spirit."

At this point it may seem as though Dr. Brewster was a fraud, taking advantage of a gullible patient. The idea of spirit possession is most definitely *not* a part of psychiatric training and normally a psychiatrist does not use exorcism as a regular therapeutic technique. But Marie firmly believed in the existence of an evil spirit possessing her body. If the doctor told her it wasn't true or that her belief was further proof of insanity, she would have rejected his care. She needed to be believed just then. She needed the doctor to deal with the problem as she saw it, not as it really existed. Only after he did that would she be willing to listen to a more rational approach to getting better.

Dr. Brewster was solemn as befit the rite of exorcism. He took an ashtray from the nurses' station and explained to Marie that since it was glass, the evil spirit could be forced to enter during the rite of exorcism. Then it was only a matter of discarding the ashtray to banish the spirit completely and forever.

How Dr. Brewster managed to keep a straight face, I'll never know. Looking back on the incident, it seems quite foolish. However, at the time Marie was absolutely convinced that she was possessed and Dr. Brewster's technique made her feel as though he was taking her seriously. This was the first big step in developing trust in him, so essential if his normal therapeutic techniques were to work.

Marie sat on a chair, clutching the crucifix, and Dr. Brewster held the ashtray over her head. "Above your head," he said, "is a glass container. I command whatever evil spirits are residing within Marie to leave her body and enter this glass container. In the name of God, the Son, and the Holy Ghost, evil spirits, leave Marie; leave Marie in peace. I command you, spirits, leave Marie! By all that's holy, leave

Marie. Leave Marie in peace and depart for wherever you go. Wherever spirits go, go there and leave Marie."

During this time Marie was sweating and straining her body as though working to expel something within. As the doctor finished speaking, Marie relaxed.

"I don't feel it anymore, Dr. Brewster. I think it's gone."

"Yes," he said, slipping the ashtray into his pocket. "All the evil spirits have gone into the glass and I will throw it into the river on my way home. The evil spirits won't trouble you again."

The doctor did not talk further about multiple personality that night. It wasn't until their next meeting together that he again approached the subject, stressing that although Marie had rid herself of whatever evil spirits were in her, that was not the same as ridding herself of alter-personalities. Such an action could only occur through counseling. She agreed to cooperate.

There are a number of techniques used during the treatment of multiple personality. While they differ from therapist to therapist and from patient to patient, basically they involve learning one's past and coming to grips with the events which took place. I developed my form of insanity as a means of mentally fleeing the rape by my father. The horror of that event lay buried in my mind. Even worse, the memories of each alter-personality were different, and Marie, who Dr. Brewster thought was the "real me," only had partial knowledge of her life as it was led after that initial mind fragmentation.

It was quite obvious to Dr. Brewster that Linda was the most dangerous personality within my head. It was Linda who became violent and Linda who tried to destroy my body. Therefore, it was important to get rid of Linda first.

One approach to treatment was to hypnotize Marie, then ask her to raise her fingers at every age when Linda was either created or reinforced through some traumatic event. He counted forward, starting with birth, then one year of age, two years, etc. A finger was raised when he reached the number five, for example, for that was when Linda came out during the rape. The finger was raised again and again as Dr. Brewster chanced upon each of the years when unusual trauma occurred.

Once Dr. Brewster knew the years involved, he would hypnotize Marie at each session and take her mentally back to the year when a trauma occurred. Then he would call out the personality who experienced the event and talk with her about what was happening. He would talk with her as though the event were recent and help the personality to understand what really took place. Often he found himself talking with a child and having to phrase his words so that a child could understand him.

I remember one therapy session when I was age-regressed to the time Marie found herself in the ranch house after the couple had adopted her. "Where are you, Marie?" asked Dr. Brewster.

"I don't know. I've never been here before." Marie sat on a chair, her knees curled up to her chest, her arms encircling them. She was under hypnosis and, though her eyes were open, her mind was reliving the experience of many years earlier. When she looked about the room, she was again seeing the ranch house.

"The room's so big," said Marie. "It's not like Grandmother's house."

"Do you see anything you remember? Any toys or people you know?"

Marie looked all over the room, then said, "No. I'm afraid. I want my mommy here. Where's Mommy?"

"She's not here right now, but there's no reason to be afraid."

"I hear voices over there," she said, pointing toward a filing cabinet. In her mind, she was actually in the ranch house, pointing toward the kitchen. "It sounds like Miriam and Al." Her face brightened and she cocked her head to one side, listening intently.

"Can you see them?"

"No, they're over there. Through the door." Marie began shifting her body on her seat.

"What are you doing now?"

"I'm trying to go see them, but my feet don't work. I can't stand up. What's wrong with me? I used to walk. I used to walk before..." Her face paled and she looked frightened.

"Perhaps if you crawled over there."

"Yes. Yes, I can do that." She smiled.

Dr. Brewster continued talking, discussing the adoption and why Marie wasn't living with her mother and grandmother. Each trauma was handled as it arose, freeing Marie's mind from yet another hindrance to her getting well.

Other techniques were used, all aimed at getting me to remember my past and come to grips with it. I began keeping a notebook of information about my life, putting down events as I remembered them. Often I would write my current feelings, fears, and beliefs, then hand the doctor the paper rather than trying to relate the information verbally. He would read what I had written and talk with me about it. The events were too painful for me to express orally, but I found I was able to relate them in writing and this was fine with Dr. Brewster.

When Marie was ready to return home from the hospital, she was afraid of what she would encounter. Although she still refused to face the reality of multiple personality, she was very slowly beginning to change. She was learning bits and pieces of her life, gaining an understanding of a tiny portion of the existence that had previously been lost from memory. Somehow she dreaded returning to the existence in which she had been living where she constantly feared for her sanity.

As soon as Marie entered the home she shared with Len and Tina, she knew it was a mistake. She sensed evilness all around her, the same kind of feeling she had had when Dr. Brewster performed the "exorcism." Trying to refrain from panic, she quickly dialed the doctor. He told her he would be right over.

Knowing that Marie was feeling the same way that she had in the hospital, Dr. Brewster grabbed an empty jar before leaving the house. When he arrived, he took it from his pocket and told Marie he was going to teach her how to mentally clean her home of all the negative emotions she felt. "Focus on the jar," said Dr. Brewster, "and fill it with the negatives you feel in this room. When you feel you have accomplished this, imagine a white beam of light sweeping through every corner and part of this room and the whole house. Doing this will protect you and keep the negatives away. You will be comfortable living here again."

Marie tried to do as he asked and found that it worked. It gave her a positive attitude toward life. For the first time in many months, she actually felt good about things.

Dr. Brewster also used the technique known as psychometry. Many times people associate objects with feelings and emotions. Marie liked to wear many different rings at the same time and had a large collection of wigs and clothing. In addition to her own clothes, her wardrobe contained Linda's purchases, which, of course, she did not remember buying.

Dr. Brewster started with the rings. He began talking about the feelings associated with them, and Marie realized that the emotions she felt when wearing them actually related to the times of their purchases.

"I feel tense wearing this ring. My body seems in knots

and I want to lash out at everyone who passes," said Marie.

"When did you get it?" asked Dr. Brewster.

"Drugs . . . I was on barbiturates. I was taking them all the time. I was always yelling at Len and Tina."

"Wearing this ring reminds you of that period in your life, a period you should be putting behind you. That's why it's important to get rid of it."

"That won't be hard. I feel like it's bringing out the worst in me. Who needs it?" Marie set the ring aside.

"This ring makes me happy," said Marie, smiling as she closed her hand around a different piece of jewelry. "I feel high with it. Not drunk or anything. Just like I could go out and conquer the world."

"Do you recall when you got it?"

"Yes, it was just after I completed the hospital work part of my nurse's training."

Then Marie thought about her wigs and clothing. She realized that her emotions were affected by the different ones she wore. In some cases, she recalled that items were purchased during low periods. Other times, when the clothing made her intensely upset, she couldn't remember buying the items at all. Actually they had been purchased by Linda, and it was this alter-personality's attitude at the time which she was sensing now.

It was around this period that Marie had an experience I still don't understand. It may have been real and it may have been a dream.

Marie was lying in bed with her eyes open. She felt there was energy in the room and seemed to see whirling dots of blackness. A piercing, whirring noise filled her ears. She felt horror and needed to hide. She seemed to be crawling away to find shelter, only there was none. The room kept changing and she felt a smothering sensation that was slowly overwhelming her.

Suddenly Marie heard a voice telling her to be calm. It

was familiar and yet she was unable to place the speaker. The voice told her to rest and fear no more. It said that her journey out of darkness had begun.

"Who are you?" asked Marie, though whether she spoke with her mouth or just her mind, she didn't know.

"You may call me Michael," said the voice.

Then another figure seemed to enter the room. It was hooded and menacing. Suddenly Michael took on human form and grappled with the hooded intruder. Marie saw colors—reds, blacks, and purples dancing before her eyes. The evil, hooded figure tried to get past Michael, fighting and screaming at him, but to no avail. Michael stood firm and at last turned the evil figure away. Then a high wind seemed to come up, causing Michael's red and black robe to swirl about. The wind grew stronger, and Michael faded from view.

Was it a dream? The vision of a mind damaged by alcohol and barbiturate abuse? Reality? Marie never knew. However, this entity called Michael would later play an important role in her fusion into a normal individual.

As therapy began, it became obvious that Marie could not continue living with Len at home. He was hostile to what was happening and skeptical of her chances of getting over the alcoholism.

Marie moved into a halfway house and found it much the same as similar places in which she had lived. No drinking was allowed, and each new arrival was expected to spend the first two weeks without seeing any visitors, including family members. Len used that time to go on vacation, though he was annoyed at having to travel without his wife.

The therapy sessions were proving effective and Marie had been dominant in controlling the body. However, one day Linda took charge, found Dr. Brewster's office number in Marie's purse, and put through a call to him.

"Tell the doc it's his newest patient," said Linda when

Dr. Brewster's secretary answered the telephone. She was nervous about making the call. In one sense it was an act of defiance. She wanted to prove to the doctor that she was the strongest person living in my mind. She had control over the others and she was the one determined to triumph. She hoped the doctor might stop treatment if he realized how formidable his opponent happened to be. Yet at the same time, she worried that this man might banish her forever. For the first time in her life, she didn't know how to deal with a man.

"Hello, Marie?" said Dr. Brewster, coming on the line.

"Guess again, doc," said Linda.

"What happened to Marie?"

"I threw her in the back of the truck and killed her. What do you think happened to her. She checked us into this alcoholic place—some half-assed halfway house. I don't belong here."

"If you don't want to be there, what do you want to be doing?"

"Drinking and fucking!"

"All right," he said calmly. He never let his voice betray any emotions he might be experiencing. "Will you be keeping the appointment Marie made with me for next week?"

"Yeah, I'll probably show up. It'll be good for laughs."

"That's good. I'll expect to see you then."

The staff members isolated Linda and tried to calm her down. When that proved impossible, Dr. Brewster was called and he again talked with Linda. He told her that he knew she was upset but he still thought it best for her to stay. He told her he had to go out of town for the weekend and he would talk with her further when he returned. He asked her to at least stay at the halfway house until he got back, and she agreed, never intending to do anything of the kind.

Linda told the staff she was going to her room to lie

down. As soon as she was certain no one was paying any attention to her, she climbed out the window and jumped to the ground. All she wore was a pair of cut-off blue Levi's and a black silk pajama top, but clothes were of no concern even though there was a dense mist in the air.

The ambivalent feelings of fear and defiance toward Dr. Brewster resulted in emotions Linda couldn't handle. The only coping mechanism she knew was fleeing to drugs or the bottle. There were no drugs handy, so she decided it was time to find a way to get drunk.

As Linda walked along a highway heading into town, a young woman drove up, pulled alongside, and asked Linda if she wanted a ride. Linda got in with her. "I'm going anywhere there's some noise and booze," said Linda. As luck would have it, the woman was on her way to work as a cocktail waitress in a downtown bar.

There was $10 in Linda's purse, but after having one drink in the bar, she realized the money wouldn't last her until she could get bombed. Liquor by the glass was just too expensive. She left the bar, found a nearby liquor store, and bought a gallon jug of cheap red wine. Then she went behind some bushes and proceeded to drink it all.

Linda returned to the bar but couldn't remember her name or where she lived. The waitress who had given her a ride into town took pity on her and offered to take her home as well. Linda began pawing through her purse, looking for some identification. At last she found a piece of paper with her home address on it and handed it to the woman.

The ride to Linda's house was interrupted when they drove past another liquor store. Linda persuaded the other woman to go inside and buy two more gallons of wine for her. Then, when she got home, she gave the woman all the money left in her purse as a way of thanking her, went inside, and proceeded to drink until she passed out. Neither Len nor Tina were there and it was three days before she awakened.

When Marie regained control, she was more frustrated than ever. She and Dr. Brewster didn't seem to be able to keep her in control. She was no closer to fusion than she had been in the hospital.

Dr. Brewster put Marie into a trance and proceeded to help her create mental images which would enable her to get control of her emotions.

"Just close your eyes and move into a state of mind where you sense you are able to move emotional energies around in your body. Think of your body as a giant battery with positive and negative emotions flowing around in it. It has two terminals like any battery—an 'out' terminal, which is your left hand, and an 'in' terminal, which is the top of your head." He placed his hand on Marie's head and pushed down slightly. "However, we are often not allowed to pass out the negative emotions, so they get stored up in our body and cause us harm. But they can be moved out, and I will show you how. It doesn't matter how long they have been in there, they don't get more fixed with time. Even those from early childhood can be removed.

"Now just concentrate on moving the anger energy out of your left foot," he continued, brushing her left shoe with his left hand. "Move the anger energy out of your toes, sole, heel, and ankle, move it up through your calf and skin to your knee. Keep moving the anger through your thighs into your buttocks. Move it out of your vagina, uterus, and ovaries. Move the anger through your abdomen and out of your back, through your heart, lungs, and chest to your shoulder. Then move it down your left arm to your elbow, through your forearm, wrist, and store it temporarily in your left hand."

Then Dr. Brewster repeated the same speech, relating

it to Marie's right side. When that was done, he took an empty jar and said, "Now start pushing all the stored-up anger into this object."

The highly suggestible Marie immediately complied in her trance state. She began squeezing very hard, as though actually moving a physical object.

"Now start moving the anger energy out of this hand, through the wrist to the forearm, past the elbow into the upper arm in the shoulder, then move it over to the other shoulder, down the arm to the wrist, and down to the hand and pour it out.

"Now the biggest amount is stored up in your head. To help you, I want you to take through the top of your head all the opposite energy of hatred, which is love. Have a beam of pure white love energy come in from above to act as a counterforce to drive the anger out." He kept his right hand on top of Marie's head and cupped his left hand above her left ear as if he was pushing something downward.

"Push the anger energy out of your skull, hair, brain, ears, eyes, nose, cheeks, chin, into your neck, down into your shoulder, down your arm, past your elbow and wrist, into your hand. Now continue to push all the anger out. Once you have the flow channels started, they will continue to work."

Marie began pushing and squeezing, obviously following the doctor's mental suggestions. For several moments she worked at ridding herself of all the anger.

As Marie mentally struggled in the trance, Dr. Brewster continued talking with her. He explained that what she was doing would not prevent her from getting angry in the future. Whenever a situation arose where anger was an appropriate response, she would express this anger. However, her emotions would be limited to what was appropriate for the moment. She would no longer be troubled by anger stored in her emotions from previous experiences.

Dr. Brewster had found that multiple-personality patients are extremely sensitive to the feelings of others. They are easily hurt and cannot seem to change. However, he discovered he could enable them to resist becoming depressed by those around them by helping them to build mental imagery which would protect them.

When Marie seemed to indicate that she was at peace with herself following the removal of the anger, Dr. Brewster asked her if she would like to learn to protect herself from being hurt so easily by others. She said she would, so while still in a trance, he had her build a mental "eggshell."

"Sit back in the chair, relax, and close your eyes," Dr. Brewster told Marie. "Now think of a beam of pure white light coming down from the sun into the top of your head. Let that beam of light fill your entire body, your trunk, arms and legs, and head. Then have it radiate from the very center of your being outward into your air space. As it does, have it push out all that is unworthy in you, all that is evil, harmful, or unwanted. Let this energy fill your entire air space so that in no way can you be outside it. Let it expand and become stronger and more brilliant so that it goes as far above your head as your arms can reach, as far to the sides as your arms can reach, as far behind you as your arms can reach, and as far below you as your hands can reach. Then, as a tomato with a soft pulp needs a skin to hold it together, start thickening up the outer surface of this energy field. Because of the shape of the human body, it will be shaped like an eggshell. Thicken this eggshell just as thick as you think you need it for protection. If things are calm and peaceful, you may need it to be only one or two inches thick. If you anticipate being around problem people, you may need it two to three feet thick. Now if you remember your biology class in school, you know that every cell in your body has around it a semipermeable membrane. This membrane is designed in such a way that food will pass through it into the cell but poisonous substances are kept out. Also, all the elements manufactured inside that are needed for the work of the cell are kept in, but all waste products are passed out. In this way a perfect relationship is maintained between this cell and all other cells. Exactly the same membrane is needed around your entire body to allow it to be in balance with other individuals.

"The first thing you need to do is to cover the outside of the eggshell with many tiny mirrors. These mirrors are designed to reflect back to their makers all negative thoughts that may be sent your way by anyone, all thoughts of malice, hatred, jealously, etc. The mirrors are 100 percent reflective, so you need add no energy to the system. Just let the negative thoughts rebound like a Ping-Pong ball bouncing off a paddle. In this way the negative thoughts will not enter your body of thoughts and interfere with the quality of your thinking. However, all positive thoughts of admiration, love, affection, and such still come right on through to improve you, help you, teach you, and otherwise benefit you. That is the first step."

The doctor continued for several more minutes, building on this image. He had Marie line her shell with a nonstick surface to help her avoid such negative emotions as hatred, guilt, and self-pity. He also explained how to retain positive emotions such as love, appreciation, and others.

When he finished with the mental imagery, he left Marie with the suggestion that she take a few moments each morning to build this eggshell anew in order to get through the day. This was especially helpful during periods when Marie had to face Len's hostility.

When Dr. Brewster finished talking with Marie, he brought her out of the trance as he had done many times before—or so he thought. But when the woman spoke, she obviously was neither Marie nor Linda. Her voice was somewhat childlike, and when Dr. Brewster asked her name, her reply was, "I don't know."

What had happened to Marie is common to many multiple-personality patients going through therapy. As they learn to cope with past problems, a new personality will be formed in the place of one or two others who are no longer needed. Rather than being a step backward, this seems to be a normal part of the progress toward fusion. In Marie's case, the new personality was named Babs, a name chosen by Dr. Brewster for no other reason than that it came readily to mind.

Babs was a self-centered, childlike individual, different from Marie, yet with all of Marie's memory. Len returned home shortly after her creation, having cut short his vacation when he called the halfway house and discovered Marie wasn't there. He took this new personality to dinner where she ordered a tremendous quantity of food, stuffing herself as though she had been starving for months.

Marie's life was difficult for Babs. She was frightened by the sound of Len's snoring as he lay by her side. However, gradually she adjusted to being a wife and mother, though she refused to have relations with Len. She had no desire for him, a fact which became increasingly difficult for him to handle.

Finally Len had enough. He confronted Babs in the kitchen and started talking about the money that was owed for the liquor store window Linda had smashed while stealing booze.

"I've got a business proposition for you, Babs," he said. She insisted he use this new name when talking with her and he agreed. He had not accepted the multiple-personality diagnosis, but he recognized that his wife could be very "changeable" and that he got along best with her when he humored her. "I'll pay your fine and the damages if you go to work for me."

"Work? What sort of work?"

"You can be a prostitute—my own exclusive whore. You fuck only me and I credit you for whatever we do. I'll give you five dollars for a plain fuck, ten dollars for a blow job, fifteen dollars for . . ."

"You're out of your mind!" said Babs, rushing to the telephone. She was shocked, frightened, and felt the need to call Dr. Brewster for help. None of the suggestions he had made for mentally protecting herself could handle this particular problem. She had to talk with him.

Babs didn't tell Dr. Brewster everything but did say that Len was suggesting they do things which frightened her. She was scared to spend the night with him, so Dr. Brewster suggested she call a friend and make arrangements to stay overnight.

Babs had no friends, so finally Dr. Brewster suggested she contact a priest of his acquaintance. The priest had a retreat which people used for meditation and to get away from outside pressures. The retreat was free to those without funds and cost whatever someone could afford if he or she had money.

Babs never did anything further to protect herself. She retreated into herself, not talking to anyone but continuing to cook and clean. Len recognized that something was seriously wrong and did not push her further.

While all this was happening with Babs, Linda had been inactive. However, one day she took control of the body, had a couple of drinks, and took a loaded rifle Len kept in the house for hunting. Everyone in the world is a blinking, blind asshole including old numb-nuts Brewster. Hell, that guy couldn't get a good hard-on if his life depended on it the way he acts around me. Maybe his wife used another man to have kids.

Brewster's better than that oversexed Len, though. His whole life is spent putting it to someone or planning how to do it. Well, he's been asking to get cut down to size for a long time. I'm going to get rid of his favorite possession. Maybe change his voice a little too. He'd be cute as a soprano.

Linda sat in a chair, the rifle across her lap, waiting for Len to come home. He was late and she quickly became bored. Finally she called Dr. Brewster, telling him of the sexual proposals Len had made to Babs. She was quite graphic, wondering if it was arousing his manhood.

"Who is this?" asked Dr. Brewster.

"Linda. Who the hell else? Do you know I've been waiting all day for Len to get here?"

"Why is that?"

"Because I'm going to shoot his balls off," said Linda, giggling. "I just haven't decided whether to blow them off when he walks in the door or wait until he's asleep."

"Doing that would be very bad, Linda," said Dr. Brewster. "You'll kill Len if you try to do that."

"I'm not going to kill him. I told you, I'm just going to blow his balls off. He'll go around with a voice higher-pitched than a canary's song."

"Take my word for it, Linda. I'm a doctor and I know that if you shoot him in the groin, he's going to die. You'll end up in jail doing fifteen years to life."

"Shit, it would be worth it just to see the look on his face when he discovers his screwing days are over."

While Dr. Brewster continued talking to Linda, the front door opened and Len stepped inside. Fortunately for him, Linda was distracted by the telephone call. She didn't notice him until he was almost next to her and then it was too late for her. He grabbed the rifle and disarmed her. He was shocked to see the entire thirteen-shell clip had been loaded and realized he had just missed being killed by her.

Shit, thought Linda. I'll have to get him later. She receded into the mind and let Babs have control of the body.

Babs looked at Len and then at the telephone receiver she was holding. She had no knowledge of what was happening.

She handed the receiver to Len, looked startled when she saw he was holding the rifle, then walked out of the room.

Len discovered it was Dr. Brewster on the telephone. He asked what his wife had been saying and Dr. Brewster gave him a general rundown. When he was through, Len was shaken by the close call he had had and wondered when, if ever, his wife would behave like a normal woman.

Linda also came out once to get drunk. Sara Carlson, her probation officer, found her drinking one afternoon, a violation of probation. She grabbed the glass Linda was using and dumped out the liquid in a desperate effort to stop the drinking. Linda responded by grabbing the jug, rushing to her room, and drowning herself in alcohol. She sat down, held the jug to her mouth, and poured it down her throat without taking a breath. She counted thirty swallows before passing out.

Sara arranged for Linda to go to the hospital emergency room. Once it was certain she would be all right, Linda was transferred to the mental ward.

Dr. Brewster recognized the fact that his patient was incapable of being without supervision. Linda was too strong to let Babs live anywhere near a liquor store, as she was doing both in the house she shared with Len and in the halfway house. He decided to arrange for a different type of treatment facility for her.

Claremont was the name of a commune started by a devoutly religious woman who believed that living a simple Christian life, working the land, and staying alive, much as the pioneers had done, was the best way to rehabilitate alcoholics, drug addicts, delinquents, and the like. She owned land in a wilderness area as well as a building that had many cell-like rooms for sleeping and a large gathering area where the members met during mealtime. Everyone farmed, hunted, and harvested crops, selling the excess for additional money. Some of the people planned to live in the commune for the rest of their lives. Others, like Babs, needed a spartan life-style on a temporary basis in order to have time to meditate on their probelms and find new ways of coping when they returned to the city.

Therapy had been going on continuously for quite a while. But the trip to the commune marked the beginning of a break in treatment. For the next several months my alter-personalities were to be deprived of face-to-face contact with Dr. Brewster. There would be contact through letters and telephone calls, and bits and pieces of my past would begin to emerge in the mind, but overall, the situation resulted in mental deterioration. For example, Babs receded and Marie returned.

Something positive did come out of the commune experience. Marie and the other personalities finally came to accept the idea of multiple personality. They each recognized that others were living parts of what should have been one person's existence. Yet none of them knew their own roles. Each thought she was the dominant one—the personality who would survive.

It was also during this period that Michael began appearing to Marie more frequently. Sometimes it was late at night, in much the same manner as the first appearance. Other times it was more like a voice in her head, giving her advice.

It was many weeks before Marie and Dr. Brewster decided to determine just what the Michael experience meant. Marie was again hypnotized, and Dr. Brewster asked to speak with Michael.

The next voice Dr. Brewster heard was deeper than Marie's and unlike that of Linda or Babs. The exact dialogue is not in my memory. Michael was a personality or entity who represented the best within me. He was created to guide the fusing of the personalities into one. When he spoke to Marie, he was trying to tell her which direction she must go to get well. Often he would take over when I was able to talk to Dr. Brewster.

Michael always spoke matter-of-factly, without emotion. Marie could be crying hysterically concerning an incident which troubled her when Michael took control. Suddenly her face would become calm, her sobbing would cease abruptly, and a deep, masculine voice would speak.

"Marie can't be on her own for the next few days," he told the doctor one time. "She isn't able to cope with the pressures of daily living. She needs to be kept in a controlled environment where she is told when to go to bed, when to arise in the morning, when to wash, and when to eat. She will be unable to handle a normal kind of existence for a while."

Once, when Marie was questioning whether or not she could truly get well, she was busy working at the typewriter, totally unaware of Michael. Suddenly she looked at the paper and saw words she knew she hadn't written. They were all in capital letters, an action apparently taken to separate the writing from her own. It read:

"I AM HERE. I GIVE YOU THE WILL TO EN-DURE THE PAIN AND THE CONFUSION THAT THE OTHER ONE WILL SEND TO YOU. I AM NOW YOUR MIND. I CONTROL YOU. GROW, GROW STRONG, AND WE SHALL WILL THE WINNING TOGETHER. FOR WE HAVE ALWAYS BEEN TWO, THOUGH YOU KNEW IT NOT YET . . ." It was signed "MICHAEL."

A variation of Michael has been found in a number of multiple-personality cases. By some definitions he is an inner self-helper. Others, who feel there is a religious aspect to the experience, feel he represents the way God talks with each person on earth, if we will only listen. No matter what the truth may be, it was Michael who proved the biggest help in bringing the personalities into a single, emotionally stable individual.

Marie left the commune in November of 1974, feeling better about herself as a result of the experience. She had enjoyed the commune, and the period of enforced sobriety had helped her improve her thinking.

Len drove to get Marie and the two of them had sex together for the first time in weeks. Although Marie found nothing strange about it, other than a degree of reluctance about going to bed with him, Len said that it was like having relations with someone he had never known before. She was changing and it was affecting their intimacy as well as other parts of their relationship.

Linda took control of the body after Marie had been back just a couple of days. She immediately went on a binge, ending up in the detoxification ward, sleeping off the drunk.

The binge cost Marie her freedom. Sara Carlson would have nothing more to do with communes or psychiatric treatment. There was only one way to handle an alcoholic parole violator in her mind. Marie was sent to the state penitentiary for women for a ninety-day hold.

Marie kept in contact with Dr. Brewster during her stay in Frontera. They sent letters back and forth, Marie using the letters as a way to come to more of an understanding about herself. One said:

My so-called recovery will be a tedious putting together of scraps of old and new information. As in most learning experiences, it will be at first slow and, perhaps on the surface, nonproductive. But I believe I have made the breakthrough at last. I try fitting the pieces together, and by honestly gaining meaningful clues, I feel I can answer, and then live with this puzzle called life. I'm sincerely trying to bring some order back, out of the original chaos.

During the next three weeks Marie wrote as much of her life's history as she could, mailing it to Dr. Brewster to give him a better understanding of the past. She covered incidents not discussed during therapy and provided him with an overview of her existence from the time she was a small child. She still knew nothing of the rape, however, nor of the original "me" buried so deeply in the mind.

There was also a deep depression evident in the writing. In another letter she said:

Madness, considered antisocial and nonserviceable, is actually the ultimate retreat for the protection of me. And I find such an escape preferable to the past. In retrospect I would that I could have done better with my life. But, on the other hand, death might well bring the ultimate happiness . . ."

When the time in Frontera came to an end, Sara Carlson was anxious to keep Marie from returning to her old life. She wanted her to enter a rehabilitation program that would keep her away from husband, child, and Dr. Brewster. She claimed that it was the only way to keep her from liquor, even though Marie pointed out that she could have gotten drunk in jail at any time she wanted. Contraband alcohol was readily available.

A hearing was held at the courthouse with the judge, Marie, Dr. Brewster, and others directly involved all present.

Dr. Brewster, Marie, and the judge adjourned to the judge's private chambers for an unusual meeting. Dr. Brewster hypnotized Marie and brought forth Michael who discussed Marie's problems. Michael was able to explain Marie's feelings as well as giving her present mental state. He described what problems would be encountered with the different types of placement under discussion.

"Marie is very weak right now," said Michael. "She is frustrated by the way she has been treated by Sara Carlson. She resents the distrust and hostility Sara shows her. She is liable to drink as an unconscious way of fighting back at the woman."

Michael later said, "Marie can benefit from living in a controlled environment but she does not belong in jail. She is not a criminal. The actions which brought her into courts were those of Linda whose power weakens as Marie comes to understand her past."

The end result was that Marie was placed in a residential treatment program for alcoholics. Unfortunately, the judge decided to let the probation department handle the matter and that meant Sara Carlson. Sara saw to it that it would be several more weeks before there was any chance of Marie's returning to regular therapy with Dr. Brewster.

Marie was returned to jail where she was overwhelmed by depression. A few moments later, Linda took charge. Linda found a bobby pin, spread it apart, and used the end to split open her arm and dissect a vein and artery. The staff caught her, however, and she quickly returned the body to Marie who, according to a letter she wrote to Dr. Brewster, was abused and searched by the staff.

> ... I was strangled, shackled, and given a digital examination on the floor in full view of the trustees and deputies while the matron spread-eagled my legs. What else can be left of my pride? I prayed in desperation for God to deliver me from the knowledge of life.

She was placed in the "blue room," the isolation cell. All her clothing was removed. She commented in that same letter:

The sixteen hours of darkness in a pit, isolated with no way to even communicate for the last five days, will burn in my heart always. Even life in an asylum must be better.

While Marie was in the county jail, Michael communicated with Dr. Brewster. Marie would be writing letters and Michael would take control long enough to send him a special message. He would explain what was happening with Marie's mental state, Linda, and the others. He also answered questions Dr. Brewster sent to Marie. Even under the worst possible circumstances for recovery, my mind was beginning to knit together, with Michael orchestrating as best he could.

By the middle of summer, treatment with Dr. Brewster was again resumed, and at last Marie was getting real therapy. The sessions went on as before, the blacked-out holes of my life gradually being filled in with facts and experiences.

Marie was placed in the psychiatric ward of the hospital, where Dr. Brewster could work with her daily. She was closely observed by the staff, as were her personality changes, which were coming less frequently. Each day she seemed to bring new dimensions to her understanding and ability to cope. Even Len noticed the changes, though he remained hostile to the therapy. He seemed to feel that he would lose his wife if she got any better, and he still wanted to think that her love for the bottle was all that was wrong.

Four months before I was cured, Marie was sitting in a semidarkened room, reading and meditating. Suddenly the name Christina came into her mind. It was a name she had never heard before, yet a name that was also familiar. She knew it was significant somehow and mentioned the fact to Dr. Brewster. However, neither of them had any idea just who Christina might be.

Len was questioned about the name Christina, but he had not heard it either. He knew his wife by the names

Linda and Marie. She had never used Christina in his presence, nor had Al or Miriam. She had insisted upon the
other names for so long; "Christina" had never come up.

The therapy continued, with Michael periodically discussing the case with Dr. Brewster when Marie was hypnotized. He warned the doctor that there were major changes
going on and soon Marie would be struggling for total control of her sanity.

It was late afternoon in early autumn when everything
began coming to a head. A man in the hall of the mental
ward was yelling, "You no-good tramp! Who are you putting
on the show for? The doctor knows what a tramp you are!"
Marie was in her room when she heard the noise and, for
some reason, thought it was her husband, Len, who was
yelling. She came rushing from her room, screaming: "Make
him shut up! Shut him up! Stop it! Do you hear me? Stop
it!"

Then Marie saw who the man really was and returned
to her room. She fell to the floor, crying.

I've got to stop that foul-mouthed blinking, blind asshole, thought Linda. There was a pair of dull scissors in the
room, the type of scissors children are given to cut construc-
tion paper in elementary school. She returned to the hall,
looking for the man who was no longer there. She entered
one room and saw a psychiatrist sitting at the desk, talking
with an obese middle-aged man whose face was covered
with freckles. She walked over to him, screeching: "Shut up,
you son of a bitch! Shut your lying mouth or I'll kill you.
If you call me a whore one more time, I'll rip your guts out
of your fat belly! Pig! Dirty, no-good fuckin' pig, pig, pig!"

Linda stabbed at the man with the scissors, hitting him
with enough force to break the skin and draw blood. Then
she whirled and fled from the room, sobbing, "I hate them!
I hate them all . . ." She blindly returned to her own room,

lay on the floor, her mind seeming to crawl into a cave of blackness.

It's dark. It's so dark. I can see the light but I'm on the floor and it's dark in here. Mommy? Mommy? Don't let Daddy hurt me . . .

No, Daddy, no!

The memory came in a flash. It was like seeing a rerun of an old movie in my head. First there was the penis—disembodied, monstrous in size, and grotesque in appearance.

Then I felt myself being grabbed and beaten. I closed my eyes, immersing myself in the memory, screaming with each previously forgotten blow. It was as if I could feel the penetration once more. I curled my body into a ball and tried to hide under a table in one of the hospital rooms. I was screaming and crying, reality and memory blending into one.

I clutched a table leg and tried to tell myself where I was. At the same time I could feel the tearing pain that came from the thrusting penis which had entered my body almost thirty years earlier.

A nurse rushed in, stroked my arm, and tried to calm me. I told myself the rape wasn't happening—only the memory. But the memory was my reality, and I had to relive the entire experience before I collapsed, sobbing into the arms of the nurse.

Dr. Brewster was summoned and I told him what I had just experienced. We both realized that this was the key to my problems and at last I was able to face it without having to split my mind into multiple personalities. I had reached a point where I could cope with reality, no matter how painful that might be. I was getting well at last.

It was October when the end came. Michael had warned Dr. Brewster that the last inner struggle was about to take place in my mind. The doctor had no idea what that meant, but he warned the nurses to be unusually alert concerning Marie's actions.

Suddenly Marie told the nurse something was going wrong. She asked the nurse to call Dr. Brewster, then collapsed on the floor.

I don't know what happened next. It is not in my memory. Michael later said that Marie had been in hell, wrestling with evil. That is probably as good an explanation as any, for I can't supply any more details. All I know is that I began writhing on the floor, screaming and convulsing, while several nurses and a security guard tried to hold me down so I wouldn't hurt myself. This continued for five minutes, I am told, and finally slowed to a stop.

Dr. Brewster arrived and used hypnosis to call out Michael. He told the doctor that everything was moving as it should. However, he needed to take the woman called Marie to the psychiatrist's office for the final change. He said that the hospital surroundings were wrong for the rebirth. Dr. Brewster, aided by one of the nurses, complied. A guard accompanied them in case Marie became violent.

Marie moved as though in a catatonic state. She said nothing and seemed to perceive nothing. She walked but did not respond when people spoke to her.

My first sensation was of warmth. My body felt warm and relaxed, as if glowing from an inner flame that heated and comforted me. I was happy, blissfully happy, though I had no idea why.

I recognized the people in the room, yet they were strangers to me. I had returned to control my own body once again. Marie, Babs, Linda, Charlene—all were gone. In their place was the person who had retreated into my mind at five years of age. Christina Peters had been born again in a thirty-three-year-old woman's body.

I was introduced to the doctor and the nurses. I asked

about my mother and grandmother and was told they weren't there right now. As the words were spoken, I began to feel my brain flooding with memories. I saw the house where I was raised, Grandmother's home, the orphanage, the ranch . . . It was like a high-speed movie going on in my mind.

I grew tired quickly, my mind bombarded to overflowing with memories. All the events that had been the unique domain of one or another of my alter-personalities were coming together in my head. Suddenly I was aware of events that had been missing all those years.

Everything was observed dispassionately. I saw Linda's sexual adventures and accepted them without concern. I witnessed the violence Linda used against my children and neither wept nor worried about what it meant. There was too much to absorb to think about any one occurrence. Later, much later, there would be time for reflection. For the moment, I had to have the memory of my lives so I could cope as a full person who would be aware of every action taken in the weeks, months, and years to come.

The warm glow stayed with me. I felt happy, as though I was discovering the world for the first time. There was no more pain; no more misery. I was devoid of fear and worry.

I wandered the halls, exploring. I found a crayon and ran my fingers over the waxy texture, marveling at the way a bit of the color clung to my hands. I glanced about to see if anyone was watching, then stuck my tongue against the tip of the crayon to taste it. I had to explore it with all my senses.

The television fascinated me. There were images dancing around the screen like little people in a box. I asked one of the women watching it what the set was called and she stared at me in amazement. I've never seen anything like that, I told her, though that wasn't exactly true. My memory bank sent images of my alter-personalities watching a variety of programs through my mind, yet I still felt that I, Christina, had never seen it.

I touched the television screen, then began running my hand around the set, sensing its warmth against my skin. Someone told me to be careful or I would electrocute myself. I didn't understand the words but could tell he was being friendly—trying to help me. I moved away, vowing to return if I had the chance so I could touch and maybe taste the plastic.

There was a water fountain and I took a drink, playing with the spout of liquid. It was cold, wet, and beautiful. I watched the way the light seemed to dance on the stream as it made its way toward the drain. I took a sip, holding the water in my mouth so I could explore the sensation of having it traveled across my tongue, between the teeth, and over the gums. The taste was familiar, yet at the same time new. I took as much delight in it as I had once experienced with an expensive liqueur.

A plant in one office was irresistible. I had to feel the leaf, the stem, and the dirt. I rooted my fingertips in the mud, trying to experience it all.

That night I watched the sun set. I laughed and cried happily, giggling as I tasted the salt of my tears.

I was Christina Peters, the person I was meant to be, and it was great to be alive!!

11

CHRISTINA

The next several weeks were extremely trying for everyone. I had the same emotional level I had when I first receded into my mind and let alter-personalities take my place. That meant I was a thirty-three-year-old woman with the emotions and responses of a five-year-old. Everything seemed new and different and I was totally incapable of being a wife and mother.

Although much of my memory returned, there was also much I did not know. Chunks of memory would come to me at odd times without any predictability. For example, I might watch a program on television and hear mention of a scientific fact, geographical location, item of history, or some other subject. As soon as I heard the words, I could suddenly remember the subject in great depth. Sadly, the one area that I forgot after fusion was my nurse's training.

Because both Dr. Brewster and I were inexperienced in knowing what a fused former multiple patient might be like, we had a "superwoman" complex. Marie had worked so hard to recover from mental illness that it was assumed that I, Christina, would be an unusually strong individual. The reality is quite different.

When I fused, it was like being given a second chance at life. I became a child once again, with all the delights that can bring and all the testing one must face. I found I had to learn to cope with life and my emotions. I had to make decisions about right and wrong, good and bad that are normally a part of an adult's moral code. It became obvious that for me to develop the maturity that my physical years indicated I should have, I would have to work as hard as I had worked to fuse my alter-personalities into one. For example, the physiological dependence on alcohol both Marie and Linda developed was transferred to me, Christina. I was reborn, yet remained an alcoholic. In fact, I am still trying to find new ways to cope with life because I am not yet free from using the bottle as a crutch when I have problems.

There is good now, as well as the problems. For the first time in my life I know what it means to have a full range of emotions at appropriate times. Linda is gone, driven from my mind when the other personalities fused. Now when I am angry, it is appropriate to the situation and does not have the insane intensity of Linda's fury. I can also laugh appropriately and feel both sadness and love. I know what it means to feel joy and sorrow, pleasure and anger, and all the other nuances of emotions. I am able to live like everyone around me and I delight in the experience.

My problems were not wiped away by the cure. I had to pay for Linda's crimes even after I was well. Because of the alcoholism, I celebrated the fusion in the way I knew best—by getting drunk. My probation still had time to run and that was a violation. As a result, I spent the first several months of 1977 back in Frontera Prison.

My personal relationships also changed. I divorced Len. When I fused, I was not the woman he had married and it would have taken many months of courtship and learning to see whether or not we could live together as husband and wife again. So far, such effort has not seemed worth it to me.

I also found that I cared almost nothing for my daughter when I fused, though that has changed for the better. A person with the emotions of a five-year-old is totally self-centered. She cannot love another, especially not as a mother needs to love her child. However, my daughter was the one relationship I was determined to regain and keep. As I matured, I made every effort to be with Tina, to get to know her and let her know me. This constant togetherness and our mutual desire to one day live as a mother and daughter should live resulted in a deep love developing between us. We are closer today than I ever imagined possible. She continues to live happily with Len and has no illusions about my problems. However, she understands and accepts me for what I am and she is the brightest part of my new life.

Dr. Brewster refused to continue therapy with me after fusion. The doctor/patient relationship is difficult at best with psychiatry. After fusion, the multiples Dr. Brewster had aided in the past always rebelled against him. He became a father figure to them and, when their emotional growth reached the adolescent level, they wanted nothing further to do with him. Rather than face this kind of conflict, he decided to insist that they begin post-fusion therapy elsewhere. I don't know if I agree with his reasoning or not. I do know that the decision hurt greatly, though perhaps that was unavoidable.

For now I am living each day for itself. I attend group therapy sessions and read everything I can find. Since my alter-personalities had such sporadic education, I feel as though I need to catch up with all those books most people read in school, as well as the latest fiction and nonfiction. I am looking for work and seriously considering going through nurse's training again.

What of the future? Do I see a bright and blissful tomorrow? I don't know. It is too early to tell. Some mornings I awaken and feel pressured by the knowledge that I am responsible for my own support. I must constantly plan what I will do and where I will go, decisions that were once made by a number of different women living in my head.

Other mornings I awaken and the warmth I felt upon first fusing returns to me. The world is new again. I am both infant and woman and I savor experiences most adults will never know.

I can see that I am maturing a little more with each new day, covering the emotional stages of growth most people my age passed through many years earlier. What is most important to me is the fact that whatever happens, I am in control of my life for the first time. Whether I drink or not, whether I take one job or another, whether I date a man or avoid interpersonal relationships for a while, are all within my power. I live each day as a whole human being. My weaknesses and my strengths are my own, not a fragmented part of me. In therapy, Marie once wrote Dr. Brewster a note born of desperation. It read: "Tell me who I am before I die." Today I am proud to say that I finally know who I am and I have only just begun to live.